SCIENCE OF BREATH

A Practical Guide

SCIENCE OF BREATH

A PRACTICAL GUIDE

Swami Rama
Rudolph Ballentine, M.D.
Alan Hymes, M.D.

The Himalayan Institute Press
Honesdale, Pennsylvania

The Himalayan Institute Press
RR 1, Box 1129
Honesdale, PA 18431 USA

Fifth Printing, 2004

Cover design by Robert Aulicino

The paper used in this publication meets the minimum
requirements of the American National Standard for Information
Sciences—Permanence of Paper for Printed Library Materials,
ANSI Z39.48-1984.

ISBN 0-89389-151-7

CONTENTS

FOREWORD

WHAT IF YOU could hold your breath for hours, exploring whole other dimensions of being while your body appeared to be dead? What if you could heal fatal diseases in a moment, just by focusing your mind? What if you could establish yourself in a state of tranquility so deep that nothing in life could ever disturb you? This, of course, is the stuff of fairy tales; people can't really do these things. And yet adepts of the ancient yoga tradition claim to accomplish these sorts of things routinely. Of course, illiterate people from superstitious cultures will claim anything.

Then in 1970, Swami Rama, raised in a Himalayan cave and trained in the closely guarded secrets of yoga from boyhood, walked into an American research laboratory. Under the most rigorous experimental conditions, he simulated death by virtually stopping his brain waves and heart beat—and yet remained fully conscious of events occurring around him in the laboratory. Reports of the swami's abilities stunned the Western scientific establishment. Suddenly the claims of the Indian yogis seemed less like superstition and more like evidence of an extensive inner science that, in many important respects, vastly exceeds the present level of knowledge of Western physicians and physiologists.

As we embark into the 21st century, modern humanity is finally learning to appreciate the profound wisdom and practical insights of ancient peoples. Tragically, just as we are awakening to the extraordinary value of medical lore developed over thousands of years, the indigenous cultures which have preserved these traditions are vanishing forever. Yet in the cave monasteries of the Himalayas and the forest hermitages of the Indian subcontinent, yoga masters continue to transmit the techniques and understanding which have made them legendary for centuries. And the key to perfect self-mastery, these yogis maintain, is *svarodaya,* the science of breath.

Breathing is the one physical function which is both involuntary (it goes on by itself) and voluntary (we can control our respiration consciously). The staggering significance of this simple insight was obvious to India's inner explorers: the breath is therefore the key to control over the autonomic nervous system, that part of our functioning we Westerners were taught lies outside our awareness and runs entirely unconsciously. By learning to manipulate their breathing patterns, yogis gained conscious control over their brain function to an extent scarcely anyone in the West would have imagined possible—until Swami Rama walked into the lab.

At the rate at which Western medicine is advancing, it may take several more centuries before our researchers catch up to Swami Rama. He insists, for example, that the physical body is actually organized around a field of energy called the *sukshma sharira* (Sanskrit for "subtle body"), the very existence of which most Western scientists still dispute. Yet it was manipulation of this energy field which allowed Swami Rama to raise tumorous growths on his arms—and make them disappear—within a matter of hours. Can you imagine how the treatment of cancer might change if medical investigators devoted even a fraction of their research funds to exploring this field of living energy?

The Sanskrit word for life energy is *prana*. The surviving

literature of the ancient peoples of Egypt and Chaldea show that they worked carefully with prana; Chinese and Japanese doctors and martial artists still work with it today. This book is an introduction to the immense subject of how yogis regulate prana through the science of breath, written in terms a Westerner can understand. The first essay explores the significance of vital energy as the active force underlying any physical organism.

Linda Johnsen

INTRODUCTION

THIS BOOK is an examination of the breath—how it integrates different levels of our being into a functional whole, the nature of the interactions occurring on various levels, and some practical methods for modifying these interactions. The scope of discussion is vast, ranging from the physical movements of the chest and abdomen to the functioning of internal organs, to the subtle play of energy flow and how it affects the mind. Precisely because its ripples influence so many human functions, a thorough understanding of the breath provides a powerful tool for expanding our awareness of the various dimensions of the body and mind. It is also useful as a therapeutic modality.

The importance of the breath can best be appreciated by observing some of the mind's properties, for the mind tends to filter many events out of conscious awareness in order to avoid a confusing barrage of sensations. This allows it to focus on the more significant changes. In other words, a new pattern of thought or a new activity initially attracts much conscious attention, but with frequent repetition it becomes unconscious and habitual. For example, walking is effortless for an adult; it requires little or no conscious attention although the conscious mind can easily intervene if necessary. However, the process of integrating the movements of walking into the mind took years of trial and error before it became habitual and could be relegated to the unconscious.

The internal organs (for example, the heart, kidney, liver) respond in a similar manner. Biofeedback research has shown that some of the physiological activities of these organs, previously labeled involuntary, can be consciously controlled with training, although much practice is usually required to become proficient in consciously controlling these organs.

Breathing is unique as a physiological function because feedback signals from the lungs and from oxygen and carbon dioxide in the blood offset the rate and depth of breathing, and yet the act of breathing itself is an act of voluntary muscles. For example, depending upon one's proficiency in dealing with the breath, the rate and depth of breathing can be altered, but involuntary reflex activity limits the degree to which this can occur. These reflexes act as safeguards, and are especially important because the need to breathe is fundamental. This in part reflects the key role played by oxygen in metabolism, for without oxygen the body cannot burn food and generate energy.

Modern science has come to understand many of the principles involved in the physical aspect of breathing, from the muscles and organs which transport oxygen into and throughout the body, down to the molecular reactions of metabolism. However, the purely intellectual appeal of these complex physiological systems has limited the scientific community's concept of the breath to the physical level only, even though the most casual reflection indicates that the significance of breath extends beyond its purely metabolic functions. For example, our personal experience suggests that there is a relationship between emotions and the breath, for intense emotional states appear to be associated with changes in breathing. The sob of grief and the trembling breath of anger are common examples. In addition, physical stimuli such as pain and exercise can act to change both the breath and the emotional state.

Once these observations are studied, a whole series of questions arises: What is the nature of the relationship between the emotions and the body and breath? What is the underlying vehicle? Does the breath interact with other realms of the mind? Can emotional and physical states be altered by changing the breathing patterns?

These are some of the questions which *Science of Breath* addresses. Each chapter develops one aspect of the central thesis that the breath is the link between the body and mind, and the authors weave together the diverse scientific discoveries of the West and the rich experiential insights of the East into a thorough and balanced exposition. After the basic tenets of the book are outlined in the first chapter, Dr. Alan Hymes presents the physiology and anatomy of the lower respiratory tract from an unusual perspective, and examines the physiological and psychological effects of various breathing habits. A discussion of the nose (an oft-maligned but rarely understood organ) and the upper respiratory tract follows in a chapter by Dr. Rudolph Ballentine. Here, this portal is examined in terms of the preparatory functions it exerts upon the incoming airstream and the complex pattern of nervous activity and energy flow which this evokes. In the final chapter, Swami Rama describes the vehicle for the body/mind interface: *prana*. According to the ancient yogic texts, prana is the most subtle unit of energy. Swami Rama discusses its organization into a pranic sheath, or energy field, which underlies the physical structure and functioning of the body and which is potentially under the control of the mind.

The goal of *Science of Breath* is to present theoretical knowledge regarding the breath in such a way that it can be applied as a tool for personal growth. To this end, a series of practical exercises and techniques for systematically working with the breath and controlling the flow of prana is described in detail. These serve to expand breath awareness, for as we observe the way in which we use our breath, various unconscious breathing habits are identified and replaced with more beneficial ones. Just as a child overcomes his clumsiness by becoming aware of his body and learning to walk, so does breath awareness gradually bring breathing under greater conscious control.

As the breath is the link between the body and mind, it can intervene in the activities of either level. With increased awareness and control of the subtle aspects of breathing, these interventions can affect deep physical and psychological changes. *Science of Breath,* then, opens up new avenues of being to the conscious mind, providing a powerful tool in the pursuit of truly holistic health and personal growth.

John Clarke, M.D.

CHAPTER ONE

WHY BOTHER WITH BREATH?
YOGA AND THE BODY OF ENERGY

MANY READERS will be surprised to find a whole book devoted to the subject of breathing, for the study of breath has not received much attention in Western medicine. In a letter to the editor printed in a well-known medical journal, a physician was complaining about the time and money wasted on research in trivial areas. "The next thing you know," he lamented, "someone will be writing a book-length dissertation on 'How to Breathe'!" He couldn't imagine a subject more trifling or a process more obvious than breathing.

Of course, breathing is a vital process. If you don't breathe, you don't live, so everyone will agree it's important in that sense. Yet most of us would say, "Either you're breathing or you're not. If you're breathing, there's no problem. If you're not breathing, you're dead, so you're not having any problems either."

Perhaps it's not that simple. In the Eastern traditions there have long been those who would spend decades studying the breath. In fact, there are entire monasteries where most of the focus centers around breathing, and it is said that many of the so-called miracles performed by yogis are based primarily on control of the breath. But why would so much emphasis be placed on an ordinary, everyday process like breathing?

The Mind/Body Problem

Our difficulty in understanding why breathing might be so strategic stems in part from our Western way of looking at the world. Our perspective is based primarily on the study of material phenomena. We take solid things and analyze them physically and chemically. Our laboratory science is based on the measurement and manipulation of matter. Our physicians are trained in anatomy and physiology. Our philosophy is basically materialistic.

In a similar way, our approach to understanding the human being is primarily physical. It's essentially based on the study of the body, the part we can touch, the measurable aspect of our being. The scientific studies we feel most comfortable with are those which treat what is objectively observable. When our research strays from the world of material objects and attempts the study of phenomena beyond the reach of our senses, we begin to feel a bit less sure of ourselves, and the question inevitably arises, "Is this really scientific?"

These doubts about the scientific validity of nonphysical studies are especially evident with respect to research in psychology, yet the mind is obviously another real level of our existence—one with which we cannot avoid coming to terms. The contemporary Westerner's interest in the mind is equaled only by uncertainty about how to approach it. It can't be dissected or measured or put in a box. It can't be put on slides and viewed under a microscope. It can't be tested with electronic instruments.

Yet our subjective experience assures us that there is such a thing as the mind and that it is important. We are all aware of our thoughts; we are aware that something is going on inside, and we admit, however grudgingly, that the workings of our mind are in some way behind most of what we do with our physical body and how we manipulate the physical world.

Yet in the West we remain confused about the relationship between the mental realm and the tangible world. How does the physical body interact with the mind? This is more than a theoretical question. The problem of mind/body interaction is one that plagues our medical scientists and baffles our psychologists. When physicians fail to alter the physical body to their patients' satisfaction, they throw up their hands and say the problem must be "psychological." When psychologists are unable to help patients reorganize their mental world, they shrug and say, "Perhaps you should see a medical doctor to make sure there's not some physical problem here." Patients shuttle back and forth between frustrated psychotherapists and puzzled physicians while the psychosomatic specialists who would understand the integration of mind and body are yet to appear on the scene.

How do the mind and body connect? Western science seems to have run into a dead end on the question. But the philosophy of the East, especially that out of which the science of yoga grew, offers a context within which some answers may emerge, for yoga includes the study of both the physical and mental realms. And these two levels of functioning constitute only a small part of the total spectrum of phenomena encompassed in the study of yoga.

Since ancient times yoga masters have spent many long hours going within themselves, studying and trying to unravel the connections existing between their various levels of existence. They discovered that, besides the physical body and the mind, there are higher levels of functioning which are also important. For instance, they uncovered and explored an area of consciousness beyond thought, a nonconceptual level of heightened and broadened awareness that could only be approached by stepping outside the arena of our everyday thinking process. The technique of inward attention which allows one to explore this level of consciousness is called meditation.

Meditation is a method used to deal with those levels of human function operating beyond the mind, what we might call "higher consciousness." Meditation is not, however, the only aspect of yoga; yoga also includes physical postures (asanas) which teach the practitioner to control, regulate, and be aware of his or her physical body. Then there are practices that have to do with the manipulation and regulation of purely mental functions—concentration, for instance. Yoga understands the human as a multileveled being, one with a series of distinct levels of existence—the physical, the mental, and what lies beyond the mind.

But in our discussion so far we have omitted mention of another important level which lies between the mind and the body, for according to yoga, the mind and the body do not directly interact. Rather, they relate to each other by way of an intermediate layer of functioning. The indifference of Western scientists to the possibility of such an intermediate state is perhaps why, for them, the relationship between body and mind is so obscure. This may be why we've been stuck with a "mind/body dualism" which seems to split our science of man asunder, leaving it in two separate and irreconcilable camps, that of the psychologist or humanist, and that of the physical scientist or laboratory researcher.

"Hard-nosed" scientists are sure that anything worthy of study is physical and material. If they wish to deal with man's actions and behavior, they limit themselves to studying and measuring the movements of the body, the production of speech, or an individual's test performance. If they think of themselves as psychologists, they prefer to label themselves behavioral scientists. The mind itself they dismiss, convinced that it is not amenable to study. This seems to be a trend of the times, though in the past decade or two the "holistic health" movement has begun to push open the door to broader awareness—a portal through which a handful of pioneering physicians and researchers have begun to step.

Fortunately in the East, and in particular among the practitioners of meditation, the relationship between body and mind has been thoroughly explored and found to constitute an intermediate link relating the body and the mind. It has its own properties and its own topography. Moreover, it is explicitly taught that this intermediate level has to do primarily with energy.

The Multileveled Nature of Man

The progress of Western science has forced us, slowly but surely, closer to this point of view. We have found it increasingly impossible to study the physical without becoming aware of phenomena that are non-physical, which we might even call "energy." We end our study of anatomy by beginning to study physiology. We end our study of physiology by beginning to study the active integration of an organism as a whole. And this level of biological functioning always involves energy.

Newtonian physicists were interested only in mechanics. They were concerned primarily with understanding how one physical body moved in relation to, and was affected by, another. In the twentieth century, however, electromagnetism has become extremely important, as has the study of nuclear forces. More and more we have come to grapple with the questions, "What is the relationship between matter and energy, between the physical realm and the realm of energy? What, in fact, is energy? If we can't see it, if it's not material, is it scientific to talk about it?" Obviously, energy is crucial. It makes us move; it makes our lightbulbs glow. Whereas our state-of-the-art machinery of a century ago burned coal to make steam and push pistons, our machinery of today has become more subtle, channeling energy through the tiniest of circuits to perform electronic miracles. How can we understand this phenomenon?

Einstein seized this question and formulated an answer. $E=mc^2$ specifies a relationship between energy and matter. It also states that they are interconvertible. Matter can be changed into energy. The most dramatic applications of this were the atomic explosions which snuffed out whole cities in Japan. Yet Einstein's formulation also states that energy can be converted into matter. The process doesn't only move in one direction.

In Sanskrit, the level of functioning involving energy is called *prana*. Advanced meditators of previous ages found that there is not only a relationship between the gross physical body and prana, but there is also a relationship between prana and the next higher level, the mind.

Intuitively, and in our everyday expressions, we acknowledge the relationship between mind and energy. At times we experience a great deal of vitality and clarity of mind, while at other times we experience a lack of "mental energy." Various schools of psychology have formulated this in more precise terms. For example, Freud called this energy libido.

According to ancient yogic texts called the Upanishads, the various levels of existence form a continuum—the physical, the pranic, the mental, and the higher levels of consciousness. These levels are layered, one upon the other. If the mind wants to affect the body, it alters the flow of energy or prana. If the body affects the mind, this too is accomplished through an effect on the flow of energy, which in turn has an impact on the mind.

Prana is called the vital link between psyche and soma—"vital" because energy is the very basis of life and vitality. When a person dies, the energy leaves. The body is still there, but the prana departs. Here we return to the matter of breath because breath is the vehicle for prana. When someone dies and the vital energy departs, we say that person has "expired." On the other hand, when someone experiences increased mental energy and creativity, we say that person is "inspired." We indicate through our language an intuitive recognition of the relationship between the inspiration, expiration, and the vital energy necessary for life and creativity.

Yet this vital area of our existence is neglected in the Western study of man. This is an intriguing situation when we stop to think about it, for if it is true that breath influences both body and mind, then the rhythm and the rate of the breath would reflect not only one's physical condition, but would also help to create it. It would be an important indication of one's emotional and mental state. Therefore, what is going on inside a person could be judged from his breathing. And this is exactly what happens. Yogis sometimes appear to "read minds" simply by observing the quality of a person's breath.

Constantly confronted with this rather obvious information, it is bizarre that we continue to ignore it. Here is something that takes place continually in the plain view of everyone, giving away the essence of our physical and mental states, giving away our secrets, so to speak, yet no one pays attention. The most fascinating and revealing kind of information is being broadcast, but no one is receiving.

We are always busy with our thoughts, which we shove around like bric-a-brac in our head. We regard them as our most intimate treasures, no doubt because our overwhelming preoccupation is with the material world, and thoughts are the means by which we consciously process our experiences and interactions with the universe outside ourselves.

Yet if we were to become aware of prana and study it, we would find it is just as complicated as the body and almost as complicated as the mind. There are, for example, different qualities of energy, different patterns through which energy can flow. These vary tremendously, both qualitatively and quantitatively.

In the Upanishads, the pranic level is described as a second body within the physical body called the "vital sheath." The Upanishads say that it takes on the shape of the physical body. If we were able to look at one another, seeing past each other's physical body, we would perceive a subtle body instead, a body of energy.

Not only is matter being pushed around through the veins and arteries and respiratory passages of our body, but changes in energy states are also taking place. Energy is being consumed in one place and produced or stored in another. It is being shifted from this point to that, so we might say there is an "energy flow." If we could stand back and look at this continually shifting picture, we would be able to map out an overall pattern of flux. Even though most of us are not able to do this, we can still understand that something of this sort is actually constantly happening.

This inner energy flow is such a delicate and intricate thing that some experts have spent their entire lifetime in its exploration. In the ancient literature of the yoga tradition, entire books have been written on the subject. These texts describe five major forms of prana, each having its own function. The pranic sheath has an extremely complex anatomy, composed of pathways called *nadis* through which the subtle energy flows.

Next arises the question of how this pranic body is regulated so that we might see whether there is some possibility of developing the ability to consciously control it. Many variables have an impact on the pattern of energy flow, yogis claim. If one contracts a muscle of the arm, the overall flow changes to accommodate this. The one function which has the most central and strategic impact on the flow, however, is that of respiration. Breathing brings in oxygen for fuel and energy exchange. Its rate and rhythm, its course and depth, all have an effect on the way the body is energized. This determines whether energy comes in frequent, short bursts or in long, more gradual waves which establish a pulsating pattern of energizing the physical body and mind. If we were to study this pattern in depth, we could derive a wave form which would describe both the frequency of energizing inputs as well as their amplitude in any particular individual at any particular time.

The flow of breath, then, is constantly helping to shape the pattern of energy flow that underlies and sustains the physical body. If we can grasp the significance of this, if we can understand the crucial way in which the energizing effects of the breath support the metabolic processes of different parts of the body, we can begin to understand how the physical aspects and activities of our body are created by and dependent on the process of breathing. With each breath, energy flows through the body in waves, constantly shaping and restructuring the pattern of energy which comprises the pranic body.

If we look at physiology from this point of view, we begin to realize that the material body, which we have tended up to this time to regard as primary, is in fact secondary to an inner field of energy even more fundamental than itself. The flow of energy creates and sustains the tissues of the body, and if the energy pattern changes sufficiently, the physical body changes also. If the energy pattern is altered drastically enough, the body can be completely transformed, for better or worse.

People's bodies do change, but they usually change in minor ways. This may be, in part, because their characteristic pattern of energy flow is set and self-sustaining since breathing habits tend to be deeply rooted in one's physiology, which has a momentum of its own.

However, when individuals sit down and deliberately begin to work with the breath, they gradually begin to see changes in the way the body functions and even, in some cases, in its appearance. The same thing happens when people endure life experiences that have tremendous effects on the way the energy flows. A shock or injury, or other trauma of some sort, may result in a change of posture or an alteration in the way the internal organs operate. Individuals may lose weight, for instance, or their complexion may change, or their face and its shape may be altered.

If the energy pattern shifts so that some part of the body is poorly supplied ("undernourished") with prana, then it will eventually become sick and perhaps even die. Physical degeneration or a malignancy may result. Some sort of disease process will become evident, for the tissues cannot function without the energizing force that supports them. On the other hand, if one's left leg is amputated, a sense of still having a leg may persist for a long while. There are common reports of patients experiencing pain in a leg which has been amputated. The patient may feel that the leg is uncomfortable or in the wrong position because the energy pattern around which the physical leg was structured requires some time to reorganize. Some animals are able to regenerate limbs which were lost. It would seem probable that this ability is based on the persistence of an energy flow to the area that was removed. Physical tissue crystallizes around the energy field that underlies it.

After part of a leaf is torn away, its energy pattern remains intact for some time; this has been demonstrated through Kirlian photography. If this pattern could be maintained long enough, it is possible that the missing portion of the leaf would grow back; in fact, some plants do have the capacity to regenerate in this way. Without this underlying energy field around which to structure themselves, how would cells "know" where to grow?

The same principle is evident in the animal kingdom where

we find one cell, after fertilization, developing into a complete animal or person. We have tended to account for this rather simplistically by saying that cells divide and redivide and eventually begin to differentiate. But how? How do some cells "know" they're supposed to change into neurons, some into muscle, and others into bone? Presumably, the information that guides the cell is contained in the chromosome. However, each of these cells has the same chromosomal structure. Yogis claim the answer is that there is a field of pre-existing forces around which the cells shape themselves.

If prana gives rise to the material level of phenomena, what, we must wonder in turn, controls the prana? According to the Upanishads, the *pranamaya kosha* or energy body is fashioned and governed by a still deeper and more fundamental level of existence called the *manomaya kosha* or mental body. This mental realm is even subtler than that of energy and still more difficult to identify, observe, and measure. Yet each of us experiences our own field of mental functioning.

When we consider these yogic concepts, we discover that we have in some way bridged the mysterious gap between mind and body. Such ideas are jarring to our usual way of thinking and yet somehow ring true. To understand our ambivalent response, we need to probe a bit deeper into the difference between how the yogi and the Westerner see themselves in relation to the universe.

Cosmic Breath

In this scientific era, we assume that the physical body gives rise to the mind, that the mind grows out of the body. According to this view, the fetus has essentially no mind.

After birth, thought and consciousness gradually develop. We look at the cosmos the same way. Somewhere on the primordial earth, molecules randomly fell into place and life appeared. Over millions of years, more complex forms of life evolved, and eventually there emerged a conscious, self-aware being.

But in the East, as in much of the ancient world, there has been a different, almost opposite, view. Yoga philosophy insists that each of the levels of being evolves out of the one *above* it. Out of consciousness comes mind; out of the mind comes the physical universe. Mind desired physical existence and so evolved a body in which to manifest itself.

This is a vastly different way of looking at the world. It implies that the essence of our being lies beyond the physical and mental cosmos. It implies that we are all manifestations of an almost inconceivable form of consciousness which lies beyond the grosser levels of our existence. It is from there we came and to there we will return. The entire universe flows out of that consciousness and ultimately flows back into its source, like a tide that flows in and out.

Oddly enough, some astronomers have arrived at a somewhat similar conclusion. It is the astronomer, of course, whose area of study pushes him hard up against the imponderables. His conceptualization of the geography of the universe forces him to deal with uncomfortable concepts like eternity and infinite space. Where does it all stop, and if time and space do end, what lies beyond them? Suddenly we realize that human rationality is a poor tool with which to measure cosmic reality.

Many astronomers today believe that the galaxies and planets are pulling apart from each other, that the space between celestial bodies is expanding due to an explosion from a dense center. This is the "Big Bang Theory," which also holds that after a certain point of expansion, the cosmos will begin to contract and all the planets, stars, and galaxies will be pulled back into yet another dense center—from which it all explodes again.

The process, then, is a familiar one of expansion and contraction. In a sense, it is nothing more than a cosmic inhalation and exhalation. All the levels of our existence can be seen as functioning harmoniously if we grasp the basic phenomenon of expansion and contraction, the "cosmic breath." On one level we manifest, we become people. We become physical, and then we return to consciousness. Hence it is that one can spend decades, or even a lifetime, delving into the subtleties and implications of the process of breathing.

Developing Awareness of Breath

How to develop control over the pranic level of one's being seems deeply mysterious or occult to us in the West. Turning to the insights of the East, we find this is not actually so. According to the yogis, the principles of prana are simple and scientific. Training in the science of breath is time-consuming only because our culture and habits have led us away from a fine-tuned level of self-awareness. However, awareness of the breath can easily become a constant part of the way we function, act, feel, and think.

Consider your left leg. Ordinarily, of course, you are not particularly worried about your left leg. At the moment you are probably not thinking, "Oh, where shall I put this leg next?" or "My gosh, when I get up am I going to be able to remember how to move it?" When you walk you generally don't have to stop and think, "Now, the left comes after the right, the right comes next, and then the left again, and I should remember to lift the toes so they won't drag on the ground." You rarely think about where exactly your left leg is, and yet you don't worry that you might have misplaced it. In a way it really is amazing that you can sit there reading this book, interact with the people around you, listen for the telephone, and still keep up with that leg.

This is possible because for years and years you've been using your legs. At first, you may recall, it wasn't so easy. It took several years for us to get it right. We started trying to put the leg, or at least the foot, into our mouth and making interesting discoveries along the way: we could wiggle our toes and feel a sharp pain if we bit into them. After a great deal of trial and error, however, we learned to walk, and before too long, we didn't even need to think about it.

It might be helpful to look at the breath in the same way. It's a system we've got running on automatic now, just like walking. Yet the breath is also something of which we can be constantly aware. Yogis who are masters of *svarodaya*, the science of breath, claim to be aware of every breath they take.

We come now to the most crucial point of all, the key to yoga science. Breathing is the only physiological process that can be either voluntary or involuntary. Individuals can breathe consciously, making the breath do whatever they wish, or they can ignore it, and the body simply breathes on its own. The body can't operate without breath, so if conscious control of the breath is abandoned, then some unconscious part of the mind reflexively begins to function and starts breathing for us. In this case, breathing falls back under the control of primitive parts of the brain, an unconscious realm of the mind where emotions, thoughts, and feelings, of which we may have little or no awareness, become involved and can wreak havoc with the rhythms of our breath. The breath may become haphazard and irregular when we lose conscious control of it.

The same thing, of course, can happen with your left leg. Sometimes people develop problems with their feet because of the way they use, or rather misuse, them. If you neglect your left foot, then instead of sensing, "Oh, there's too much pressure on the lateral insole" and making an adjustment, you simply go on walking as usual. Eventually the foot becomes twisted and distorted. Then you pay a podiatrist a hefty fee to show you some foot exercises, slowly bringing the foot back into your awareness so it can begin to function properly and heal.

The same thing happens with the breath. It can either be allowed to run haphazardly and create havoc in the body and mind, or it can become a part of your constant awareness and be harmoniously coordinated. And once the breath is integrated into your awareness, you'll wonder how you ever got along before.

People who have been injured and haven't walked for some time may develop the habit of ignoring the lower half of their body. They live from the waist up. What's above the waist is alive whereas what's below is dead weight. As these people recover the functioning of the injured half, they go through an elaborate process of learning how to use their legs again. They have to extend their awareness back down into their legs, which requires hard work because they had mentally disavowed that part of themselves, ignoring it, cutting it off.

And here is the problem we begin to confront when we learn about breathing. We must bring back into our awareness a whole area of ourselves that we've cut off, gradually reintegrating it into our consciousness. The more we make it part of our constant awareness, the more it becomes a vital dimension of ourselves.

At that point the teachings of *pranayama* (breath control) begin to make sense. Through constant awareness and experience we discover for ourselves what happens when we breathe through one nostril or the other. We notice that when the breath switches from the right to the left nostril, there is a shift of physical and mental tone. For example, having lunch today with the left nostril open is followed by the realization that the food didn't sit as well as usual. The scriptures say we should eat only when the right nostril is open. Because the emotions are closely related to the breath, by altering our respiratory rhythm we should be able to shift emotional gears. This is something we can try out, experiment with from moment to moment. In this way the science of breath ceases to be mere theory and becomes part of practical experience, vastly enriching our self-knowledge.

This awareness comes gradually. The stage for this self-exploration is set by understanding the mechanics of prana and by the regular practice of breath awareness and breathing exercises. The result is an awakening of a whole part of ourselves that we didn't know was there before, a completely new aspect of our being to which our eyes had been closed. Svarodaya, the science of breath, opens our inner awareness to the very energy that gives us life and shapes our being.

CHAPTER TWO

RESPIRATION AND THE CHEST: THE MECHANICS OF BREATHING

Alan Hymes, M.D.

FEW BASIC physiological functions have escaped the attention of modern man to the degree that breathing has. The importance of the heart, for instance, is known to everyone, largely because of the prevalence of coronary artery disease. Similarly, preoccupation with the digestive organs is obvious from the bewildering array of commercial preparations available to treat them. In contrast, except for diseases associated with smoking, the respiratory organs have been largely ignored. Considering that anyone can readily modify the flow of breath, whereas control of other internal organs is largely inaccessible to the average person, this is all the more surprising.

Knowledge of the dynamics of breathing, however, need not remain shrouded in ignorance. By understanding a few basic principles of how the respiratory process operates and interacts with the body and mind, one can readily gain clear and intensely practical insight into previously unknown levels of physiological and psychological functioning, for the movement of muscles to transport air in and out of the body is only the grossest manifestation of the breathing process. The effects of breathing extend to the workings of the heart and lungs as well as to subtle physiological interactions such as the molecular processes through which the body's energy production is maintained.

Cellular Respiration

All organisms—human, plant, or animal—are composed of a multitude of tiny individual living units called cells, and it is these cells and the manner in which they are organized into specific tissues and organs that form the physical body. The very life of these individual cells and therefore the body as a whole are dependent upon a continuous source of energy.

We usually think of the food we eat as supplying our energy needs in terms of a certain amount of carbohydrate, protein, and fat, but these nutrients are actually useless to the body unless they can be converted into a form which can be used by its cells. In other words, it is often said that we burn carbohydrates in the body, but what does this mean? If carbohydrate is being burned in my tissues, why doesn't my fat sizzle? Where does the smoke go? If I exercise vigorously in a dark room, shouldn't I be able to see my body glow from the flames produced by the burning carbohydrate? We often hear that the body is 88 percent water. How can I burn carbohydrate in that much water when I can't even get a campfire started when the wood is a little damp?

In a fire, energy is released in the form of heat and light. The reaction involves the burning of carbon-containing substance. If the process is efficient, the end result is the formulation of carbon dioxide, water, and ash, along with the release of energy.

The heat energy in a fire can be used to drive a machine such as a steam engine, but an automobile engine is driven by a more rapid burning process: gasoline exploding in a chamber. A coordinated series of controlled explosions in multiple chambers called cylinders turns a shaft, which in turn spins the wheels of the car.

How then does our body harness energy? Cells must have energy, but they do not run on explosions. Instead, all living organisms can be thought of as meeting their energy needs from a slow-burning furnace. This furnace releases energy from a constant supply of fuel by slowly combining it with oxygen. In a rapidly burning system, oxygen present in the air combines instantly with fuel so that a readily visible fire results. The products of this burning are carbon dioxide, water, heat, and light, and in rapidly burning systems, this reaction can be quite dramatic, such as a firecracker exploding. However, when fuel is consumed more slowly, energy is produced at a slower rate, yielding a steady flame. If the rate of burn is exceptionally slow, there may be no light visible at all. Biological systems—all living organisms—are essentially burning fuel at a very slow rate.

The fuel that we use biologically comes from the carbohydrates and fats we eat. This energy release must take place under special circumstances to keep in a form that is both useful and safe. That is why the reaction takes place in tiny subunits within the cell called mitochondria. These contain a series of specialized protein molecules or enzymes, called the cytochrome oxidase system, which transfer the energy released from the oxidation of our food to a storage molecule called adenosine triphosphate, or ATP. Found in biological systems throughout nature, for practical purposes ATP may be thought of as the basic unit of energy storage for cells. It has the ability to deliver energy within the cells of the body, which in turn maintains the chemical reactions necessary for the cells to function normally.

The actual process of respiration, then, occurs within the cell where nutrient fuel is burned with oxygen to release energy. The nose, trachea (windpipe), lungs, circulatory system, and their attendant muscles all act to transport or modify oxygen from the surrounding air to make it readily available to individual cells. Each of these organs plays a crucial role in determining oxygen supply, and therefore energy availability, to cells at various levels within the body. Consequently, a change in functioning in any one of these systems could potentially alter the course of energy production within the entire body.

The Pulmonary and Circulatory Systems

In order for oxygen to become available for use in the cell, it undergoes an interesting journey from the atmosphere through the lungs and circulatory system and finally into the cell itself.

As air is inhaled through the nose and into the chest, it encounters the main airway leading to the lungs, the trachea. This is a smooth, tube-like structure beginning just below the larynx or Adam's apple and which splits into two smaller tubes, one supplying each lung. These airways, called bronchi, branch off like limbs on a tree, getting smaller and smaller until they become microscopic in size. After about fifteen "generations" or branching levels, they terminate in tiny bronchioles, and each of these in turn ends

The Bronchial Tree

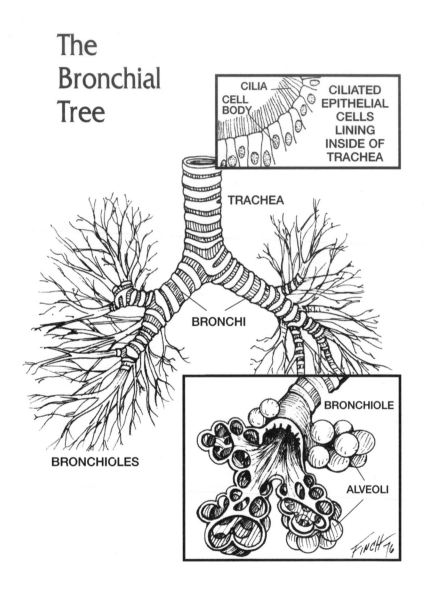

CILIA
CELL BODY
CILIATED EPITHELIAL CELLS LINING INSIDE OF TRACHEA

TRACHEA

BRONCHI

BRONCHIOLES

BRONCHIOLE

ALVEOLI

FINCH 76

in a series of very tiny air sacs called alveoli. These air sacs are so small that lung tissue actually looks solid and fleshy to the naked eye. In reality, however, the alveoli are much like bubbles. They have very thin walls—only one cell thick—and these cells, too, are very thin and membranous. It is here that the gas exchange occurs.

Surrounding the alveoli is a network of tiny blood vessels, capillaries so thin that blood cells literally have to squeeze their way through. Oxygen in the atmosphere moves from the nose or mouth down the trachea, through the bronchial system, and into the alveoli. From there, the oxygen is absorbed into the bloodstream flowing through the capillaries surrounding the alveoli.

For this process to take place efficiently, there should ideally be a balance between the amount of blood flowing within the capillaries to absorb oxygen and the amount of oxygen brought to the alveoli by breathing. The casual observer might say, "Well, that's obvious." But the physiology of the lungs shows that blood is not evenly distributed throughout the entire lung field. It is gravity-dependent, and in the upright position there is far more blood in the lower part of the lungs than the upper part. However, the free flow of gases into and out of the alveoli is greater in the upper portions of the lungs, so this process of oxygen transfer from the atmosphere into the blood is not necessarily as efficient as it appears at first glance. The degree of inefficiency can be reduced not only by compensating reflexes in the lungs, but also by the way in which we habitually breathe.

More serious inefficiencies develop if the alveoli become injured, as they do from smoking, for if the lining of the many tiny alveoli breaks down, what was once an area consisting of multiple small chambers becomes one larger pocket which appears as a visible hole in the lung tissue. When this happens, the tremendous surface area over which oxygen comes into contact with blood is significantly reduced, resulting in a condition called emphysema. It develops slowly and silently, over a period of years, because of noxious fumes taken into the lungs, destroying the delicate walls of the alveoli.

The most common cause of emphysema is cigarette smoking, and it is such a problem that several million Americans are crippled by it. All smokers have emphysema to some degree, but because of the enormous area that exists for diffusion of oxygen, in its early stages most people are not aware they have this condition while they go about their normal activities. Most people have about 300 million alveoli in their lungs. If one could flatten each of these out and lay them side by side, they would cover an area greater than an average one-bedroom apartment. It is only when this area becomes drastically reduced that people find they cannot exchange enough gas to keep up with their oxygen needs when they increase. They will notice this during exercise, for example, and feel "short of breath."

Oxygen, once it gets into the busy capillaries, can be transported by two basic mechanisms: it can either be bound by the hemoglobin molecule within red blood cells or it can dissolve directly into the blood. Practically all of the oxygen which is transported through the bloodstream is carried by hemoglobin. This molecule is composed of four protein chains attached to one atom of iron, and it is this iron atom which attracts oxygen gas and which facilitates the transport of oxygen throughout the body. When oxygen is bound to this iron atom, it turns the freshly oxygenated blood a fiery red. Hemoglobin can also carry carbon dioxide, a waste product from cells, which it picks up for the return trip to the heart and lungs. The combination of carbon dioxide with hemoglobin, along with the loss of oxygen, gives a bluish color to the blood, and this, of course, is why arterial blood is bright red and venous blood bluish.

Normally oxygen and carbon dioxide should be the only molecules which bind to hemoglobin. However, some other gases present in the environment can enter the bloodstream via the lungs and also bind, essentially crowding the oxygen out of the hemoglobin. A common substance that does exactly this is carbon monoxide, which appears in high concentrations in both cigarette smoke and automobile exhaust fumes. Having an affinity for hemoglobin that is 240 times that of oxygen, carbon monoxide quickly latches onto a hemoglobin molecule, and since the carbon monoxide removes the hemoglobin from the oxygen transport system, this results in a decreased amount of hemoglobin available to carry oxygen—or a relative anemia. People who smoke cigarettes may have from 5 to 15 percent of all their hemoglobin tied up with carbon monoxide at any given time, even if they are not smoking at that moment.

The problem actually goes further than that because carbon monoxide may also contribute to hardening of the arteries, or arteriosclerotic disease. The exact mechanism by which carbon monoxide gives rise to this disease process is not completely understood although it has been observed both clinically and experimentally. The death rate in smokers from heart attacks and strokes is approximately three to five times greater than the death rate in nonsmokers.

Once hemoglobin molecules are oxygenated, they still have to travel throughout the body in order to supply the needs of individual cells, and the driving force which propels blood throughout the body is, of course, the heart. This organ is divided into two separate functional sections. The right side takes oxygen-poor (carbon dioxide-rich) venous blood from the body and pumps it into the capillaries surrounding the lung's alveoli where gas exchange occurs. Then this newly oxygenated arterial blood is redistributed throughout the body by the left side of the heart. As the oxygenated blood approaches the cells along its route, it moves through increasingly smaller vessels to the point where red blood cells squeeze through capillaries that are the same size as those surrounding the alveoli in the lungs. This time, however, the capillaries surround cells in other parts of the body (muscles, nerves, etc.), and at this point gas exchange similar to that which takes place in the lungs occurs—but now it is between the hemoglobin and a cell. Here, waste carbon dioxide from the cell is exchanged for oxygen from the red blood cell hemoglobin, depleting the blood of oxygen and turning it blue. This newly made venous blood then travels through a series of successively larger veins, eventually going through the right side of the heart and winding up back in the lungs to complete the cycle again.

The Mechanics of Breathing

Previously, the respiratory system was discussed in terms of levels which are not readily visible to the casual observer: molecular interactions, microscopic transport, and internal anatomy. The focus of discussion now shifts closer to the body's surface in order to study the organization and action of those structures which create the driving force for moving air in and out of the body.

In looking at the body, several anatomical divisions become readily apparent: the four limbs, the head, and the torso. Each comprises a distinct anatomical unit. Since it is the torso which contains the organs responsible for movement of air into the body, as well as the other major organ systems responsible for distribution of oxygen, it is here that a discussion of the mechanics of breathing must be centered.

One can subdivide the torso into three regions: the thorax or chest, which houses the heart and two lungs; the abdomen, which begins immediately below the thorax, separated from it by a sheet of muscle called the diaphragm, and which contains the organs of digestion; and finally, the pelvis, which extends from the hipbones down to the bottom of the torso and houses the organs of excretion and reproduction. For the purposes of this discussion, the pelvis will be considered as essentially continuous with the abdomen.

Looking only at the supporting bone, muscle, and skin, with the internal organs removed, the torso can be viewed as forming a rough cylinder, slightly flattened out, so that it is wider than it is deep when seen in cross section. The bony spine, or vertebral column, which runs vertically through the back parallel to the long axis of the torso "cylinder," provides structural support for the whole torso, acting as a framework around which other tissues and organs are grouped. The vertebral column itself is composed of a number of small individual bones called vertebrae. They are stacked, one on top of the other, and are separated by discs of shock-absorbing tissue. The first twelve of these bones within the torso, the thoracic vertebrae, each attach to a pair of ribs, one on either side. The ribs all travel parallel to each other, curving in a forward and downward direction. The first ten of these join in the midline and fuse with the sternum, or breastbone, to form the rib cage. A series of small joints connect the ribs and vertebrae; this allows them to move slightly in a hinged fashion, somewhat like a curved bucket handle moves. The ribs, along with their attachments to the sternum in front and vertebral column in back, form the walls of the thoracic, or chest, portion of the body cylinder.

Because the ribs gradually increase in length of curvature from the top to the bottom of the thorax, the widest part of the thorax occurs at its lower margin. Attached to these lower ribs and to the sternum and vertebral column is a tough, flat sheet of muscle, the diaphragm, which in effect divides the torso cylinder into two smaller cylinders, one stacked on top of the other, the chest cavity above and the abdominal cavity below. The boundaries of the abdominal cylinder include the vertebral column and its supporting muscles in the back and the floor of the pelvis, both of which are relatively inflexible and fixed, and the abdominal contents which lie just beneath the surface of the diaphragm, extending partly into the chest cavity. Several overlapping sheets of muscle, extending from the ribs above to the pelvis below, form the front and sides of the abdomen.

The diaphragm, which separates the chest and abdominal cavities, is not flat in its resting position, but billows up into the chest cavity somewhat like a parachute or dome. For this reason its movements are not directly visible at the body's surface, and one has to infer its activity based on the effects its movements have on other body tissues.

Immediately above the diaphragm are the right and left lungs, and nestled between them, the heart. The lungs do not actually touch the diaphragm directly, for they are completely covered with a very thin double layer of tissue known as pleura. Normally, these two layers are in direct contact with each other, slightly moistened by a small amount of pleural fluid which acts as a lubricant, allowing the pleural layers to freely slide over each other.

The innermost pleural layer completely covers the outside of each lung, while the outer layer covers the inner surface of the chest wall and the thoracic side of the diaphragm. Since both pleural layers are in such close contact with one another, a movement of the chest wall or diaphragm will be transmitted to the lungs, and vice versa. If, for instance, the diaphragm moves downward or the ribs expand outward, the lungs will follow, expanding in the process. These are, in fact, the two main mechanisms by which air moves into the lungs.

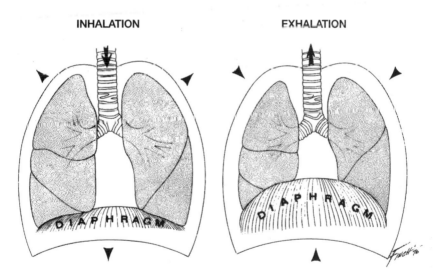

Airflow into the lungs occurs when the structures surrounding them expand and pull the lungs along with them. The resulting suction pulls air into the lungs from the upper airways to the trachea and bronchial tree, into the alveoli. This is the process of inhalation.

Thinking of the chest cavity as a cylinder again, one can produce an increase in its volume, and consequently inhalation, by one of three means: extending the diaphragmatic floor of the cylinder downward, expanding the walls outward, or moving the top of the cylinder upward. These three phases will be termed diaphragmatic breathing, thoracic or chest breathing, and clavicular breathing. As will be seen, these three phases occur in sequence when one breathes to maximum capacity as in the complete yogic breath.

Diaphragmatic inhalation, then, is accomplished by moving the diaphragm downward. How is this done? The diaphragm, like all muscles, can assume two states: an active contracted state in which the individual muscle fibers shorten or a passive relaxed state in which muscle fibers achieve a maximum length. In its relaxed state the diaphragm is shaped like a domed parachute with its rounded surface bulging upward. During contraction the remaining "slack" is taken up when the individual muscle fibers contract. The diaphragm then tends to assume the smallest surface area possible, which, since it is attached to the edges of the thoracic cylinder, flattens it from a dome to a disc. This markedly increases chest cavity volume. But as the diaphragm moves down, it decreases the volume of the abdominal cavity, so if the abdominal wall is relaxed, it moves passively outward, re-establishing the volume needed for the abdominal organs.

Of the three types of breathing mentioned, diaphragmatic breathing is physiologically the most efficient. A major portion of the blood circulating in the lungs goes to the lower portions, or gravity-dependent parts, and expansion occurs in these lower portions (although all of the lung expands to some degree). Since one of the purposes of breathing is to expose the blood in the capillaries to air, diaphragmatic breathing in the upright position is very efficient. It is also interesting to note that infants and small children use their diaphragms exclusively for breathing. Chest breathing cannot occur until considerably after birth, after the bony chest matures.

A second major way of moving air into the lungs is to expand the diameter of the thorax which involves moving the ribs around their joints of attachment to the vertebrae. A specialized group of muscles, the intercostals (Latin for "between the ribs"), performs this function. Many people have experienced these muscles as the "meat" sandwiched between the bones of barbecued ribs. These muscles exist in two layers, external and internal. The external muscles are aligned in such a way as to actually swing the ribs upward and forward, pivoting them around their joints with the vertebrae. This increases the diameter of the chest, and the lungs consequently expand, pulling air into the alveoli to fill the newly created space. The internal intercostals perform exactly the opposite function, pulling the ribs down and in, effecting a reduction in lung volume.

Chest breathing fills the middle and upper portion of the lungs with air but is not as efficient with the lower portion. When the body is upright, however, most of the blood is in the lower, gravity-dependent areas, so air is not mixed as thoroughly with blood if breathing is done by expanding the ribs. Chest breathing also requires more work to accomplish the same blood/gas mixing than does slow, deep, diaphragmatic breathing. Since more work is required, more oxygen is needed, resulting in one's taking more frequent breaths. Finally, more blood needs to circulate through the lungs, requiring more work from the heart. How much work the cardiovascular system must do, then, is directly related to how efficiently one breathes.

The third type of inhalation, clavicular, is only significant when the maximum amount of air is needed, for example, during vigorous exercise. Its name derives from the two clavicles, or collarbones, which are pulled up slightly at the end of maximum inhalation, for this movement expands and lengthens the top of the thoracic cylinder, and thus the very top of the lungs. Clavicular breathing only comes into play when the body's oxygen demands are great.

The three types of inhalation can be coordinated into one smooth exercise in which a maximum deep breath is taken. This is the yogic complete breath which has a diaphragmatic, thoracic, and clavicular phase. It is initiated by diaphragmatic contraction, resulting in a slight expansion of the lower ribs and protrusion of the upper abdomen, thus oxygenating the lower lung fields. Then the middle portions of the lungs expand, with outward chest movement, in the thoracic phase as inhalation proceeds further. At the end of inhalation, still more air is admitted by slightly raising the clavicles, thereby expanding the uppermost tips of the lungs. In sequence, then, each phase of inhalation acts on one particular area of the lungs.

After the lungs are filled to their capacity with air, how are they emptied? What results in exhalation? Relaxation. Everyone has had the experience of sighing or letting a deep breath out in a completely relaxed, passive motion. No muscles contract to push the air out. It is as if the lungs themselves are pulling the diaphragm and chest wall in. This is, in fact, what happens. The lungs act as if they are elastic, and they shrink back to their original size once the forces which expanded them are released, much as a balloon shrinks back to its normal size once the end is untied.

The reason for this elastic recoil is quite fascinating. Again like a balloon, the lung has some elastic fibers in its tissue. But, more importantly, the elasticity is related to the millions upon millions of tiny rounded pockets of cells, the alveoli. Each one of these alveoli is coated inside by a thin layer of protein-containing fluid called surfactant, which is the secret behind the lung's elastic properties, for surfactant possesses a property common to all fluids known as surface tension. This property can be illustrated by looking at a soap bubble. The walls of the bubble, being mostly water with some dissolved soap, are liquid. As one blows on the bubble, the trailing edges snap together to form a sphere while the surface layer of the soapy water exerts a force, or tension, drawing it together to assume the smallest area possible—which in three dimensions is a sphere. Surface tension then continues to maintain this round shape. For the same reason, beads of water and other liquids tend to assume a rounded shape.

In the lungs, the effects of surface tension are important, considering the large area covered by surfactant since, in order for inhalation to occur, the muscles involved must overcome the effects of surface tension in order to expand the lungs. Once the muscles relax, however, surface tension is unopposed, the lungs are drawn together, and the chest and diaphragm follow suit. The intercostal and abdominal muscles can, of course, augment exhalation, speeding up or deepening the process, but it is the lungs' ability to recoil on their own that is of crucial importance. People whose respiratory muscles—with the exception of the diaphragm—are paralyzed can still inhale and exhale without assistance, for surface tension provides sufficient opposition to the diaphragm to maintain breathing by itself.

This explains why the relaxed diaphragm billows upward

like a parachute instead of sagging into the abdomen, pulled down by gravity. Surface tension within the lungs keeps them contracted when the respiratory muscles are relaxed. This force is stronger than gravity, and the diaphragm thus remains supported, pulled upward by the lungs via the pleural layers. There are interesting differences in the inter- play between diaphragmatic motion and gravity, depending upon the posture one assumes. If the body is in an upright posture, gravity tends to pull downward on the abdominal contents, the diaphragm and the lungs, opposing the elastic recoil of the lungs and facilitating the downward movement of the diaphragm during inhalation.

When a person lies flat on his or her back, the diaphragm is oriented vertically with respect to the floor and pushes the abdominal wall upward when it contracts during inhalation, requiring a slightly increased force of diaphragmatic contrac- tion. During exhalation, gravity can then act to pull this abdominal bulge downward when the diaphragm relaxes, and the abdominal contents, no longer pushed by the diaphragm against gravity, move against the flaccid diaphragm, helping to restore it to its original resting position. Little or no mus- cular effort is needed to counterbalance diaphragmatic con- traction in this position during inhalation.

Complete exhalation beyond the position at which the diaphragm is at rest requires active muscular effort in oppo- sition to that involved in a complete breath except that the diaphragm no longer takes part. Since a muscle can only contract in one direction, a second muscle or force is re- quired for active movement in the opposite direction. Look- ing at the three phases of breathing that take place in the yogic complete breath, three opposing sets of forces are nec- essary for extreme exhalation. Therefore several muscles are attached to the clavicles, and one can clearly define muscle groups which act to either elevate or depress them for a full cycle of inhalation/exhalation. Similarly, the external intercostals are paired with the internal intercostals, each group opposing the action of the other in the thoracic phase of breathing.

There is, however, no muscle or group of muscles which are paired with the diaphragm to produce muscular contraction in exactly the opposite direction, but a set of muscles does exist which can act to achieve a similar effect. These are the abdominal muscles, four layers of muscle which crisscross each other to form the front and side walls of the abdomen. During inhalation, the diaphragm pushes the abdominal organs downward, causing the abdomen to bulge forward. As the abdominal wall contracts during exhalation, it pushes the abdominal organs upward against a relaxed diaphragm, compressing and emptying the lungs.

Breathing Habits

We have seen that the breathing process has an influence upon various levels of the organism, from subtle molecular interactions in the energization of ATP by oxygen, to the grosser physical movements which propel air in and out of the lungs. Of these levels the most visible, and the one with which we identify most closely, is the physical motion of the chest and abdomen. To breathe is before all else to move air into and out of the body, and the motion of the chest and diaphragm is the essential first step in determining the amount and manner in which oxygen is delivered for respiration.

That the quantity of air taken into the body is important is obvious. Not enough air and consequently insufficient oxygen to meet the body's energy demands will result in a reduction, or even cessation, of cellular functioning, ending in death. Less obvious, but of great importance in maintaining health, is the quality of the breathing process, that is, the manner in which air is inspired and expired. Identifying whether breathing is diaphragmatic or thoracic, continuous or interrupted by pauses, rhythmical or irregular can be of major significance in determining one's physical and emotional state. By looking at a single specific breathing characteristic or group of characteristics, we can then speak of different breathing modes or habits. Everyone has had some experience with a disruption in breathing pattern associated with pain or powerful emotions. A sob of grief, a startled gasp, and the deep trembling breaths of one in anger are familiar examples of how emotion can affect breathing. But the relationship extends beyond this, for a change in the breathing pattern can also alter an emotional state as well as effect physiological changes in the body. An examination of some common breathing habits will clarify this.

During average daily activities, most people predominantly employ a variant of either chest or diaphragmatic breathing. The maximum inhalation of the yogic complete breath can be performed for short periods of time as a breathing exercise or during heavy physical activity when oxygen requirements are high, but it is otherwise rarely encountered.

Of the various types of breathing, the one best suited for everyday relaxed functioning is diaphragmatic breathing. Here, lung expansion is focused on the lower, gravity-dependent areas of the lung where oxygen exchange can proceed more efficiently. The diaphragm performs its function well, not only in adults, but also in infants and young children where it is the sole muscle of inhalation. In addition to providing the most efficient breathing pattern, the diaphragm, as it contracts, pushes the abdominal organs down and forward, and this rhythmical massage gently compresses the abdominal organs, promoting improved circulation.

In addition to being an excellent regular mode of functioning, diaphragmatic breathing has shown potential as a therapeutic tool in dealing with several abnormalities. Essential hypertension (high blood pressure of unknown cause) has been shown to respond favorably to a daily regimen of diaphragmatic breathing. This is especially encouraging when one considers the number of deaths per year in the U.S. from heart disease alone that are associated with hypertension. Diaphragmatic breathing, in conjunction with relaxation exercises, has resulted in impressive improvements in treating anxiety states in at least one study, and this represents a mode of treatment free from the potential side effects of medications. The application of such a simple, safe, and inexpensive method as an adjunct to other therapies is an exciting one for further research.

A second type of breathing, chest breathing, occurs frequently in our society. Here chest wall movement, rather than diaphragmatic movement, is the major component of breathing. Expansion is therefore centered at the midportion of the lungs, and gas exchange is consequently less efficient than in diaphragmatic breathing. For a number of reasons, too, there is evidence to indicate that anxiety is more frequently associated with chest breathing as opposed to diaphragmatic breathing if it is employed as the major resting breath pattern. A number of therapists, notably from Alexander Lowen's school of bioenergetics, place great importance on breathing, maintaining that many people actually "freeze" or immobilize their diaphragms in an attempt to contain fears of aggression and other powerful feelings and keep them out of consciousness. Since psychoanalysts hold that emotions centered on sex, fear, and aggression have strong associations with lower parts of the body, stiffening the diaphragm can serve to isolate the associated feelings in the lower body, pushing them out of awareness.

It has also been suggested that chest breathing relates to our popular conceptions of body image. Normal diaphragmatic breathing pushes the abdomen forward during inhalation, but unfortunately a protruding abdomen is not fashionable in our society. The wide shoulders of an athlete, tapering to a thin waist, and the hourglass figure of a bathing beauty represent the epitome of popular beauty, so many people push out their chest and pull in the abdomen, keeping it tense, thereby limiting diaphragmatic movement. This could lead to an increased reliance upon chest breathing to supply the body's oxygen requirements, as well as chronic muscle tension in the chest and abdomen.

A physiological theory has also been proposed in an attempt to relate anxiety and chest breathing. Whenever we anticipate physical or emotional stress, such as a sports event, an emotional crisis, or an unavoidable accident, the body gears up its defense mechanisms and prepares to deal with the confrontation by either "flight or fight." The response is one we have all experienced at some time and is characterized by cold, sweaty palms, a pounding heart, and acute anxiety. Coordination of this response is achieved by the autonomic nervous system, that network which controls the functioning of those internal organs and tissues which do not require constant conscious input in order to operate smoothly (for example, the heart, liver, kidneys, bowels).

Anatomically and physiologically, the autonomic nervous

system is divided into two branches, the parasympathetic and sympathetic systems. The former is involved in controlling resting activities: slowing the heart rate, speeding digestion, and activating the cleansing processes of the body. In contrast, the sympathetic system regulates more active, externally directed functions such as those involved in responding to emergency situations or physical exercise. When the sympathetic nervous system is activated, the heart rate increases and blood is shunted away from the digestive and excretory organs to the muscles of the limbs, readying the body for physical activity. The balance between sympathetic and parasympathetic systems is reciprocal and determines the overall state of the autonomic nervous system at a given moment.

Breathing, also under autonomic control, becomes accentuated during the "fight or flight" response, and even where diaphragmatic breathing may have predominated earlier, chest breathing now also appears to meet the anticipated increased oxygen needs. If the anticipated event results in physical activity, the body is prepared and discharges its accumulated energy; if not, hyperventilation, in association with anxiety, is commonly seen. In this case an increased amount of air is exchanged by the bloodstream due to excessive breathing. If no physical activity has occurred to achieve a balance in gas exchange and if the "red warning lights" continue to flash in one's head, the physical symptoms, anxiety state, and excessive breathing continue. In susceptible people, this hyperventilation alone can cause a metabolic derangement resulting in irritability and/or lightheadedness, and a further increase in anxiety.

It has been suggested that by chronic chest breathing one can perpetuate or cause a state of sympathetic nervous system arousal, recreating the above situation. For this reason, studying the interrelationship between emotions, breath, and the autonomic nervous system could potentially yield valuable insights into the prevention and treatment of numerous diseases.

Still another major breathing type, paradoxical breathing, involves a combination of expanding the chest while simultaneously contracting the abdominal muscles, which pushes the diaphragm up into the chest cavity. Although the chest wall expands, increasing lung volume, the diaphragm simultaneously rises and diminishes these gains. It is immediately obvious that this cannot be an efficient way to breathe, fighting against oneself for air. Then why would anyone breathe this way?

Although breathing is partly under voluntary control, as mentioned earlier, it is also regulated by the autonomic nervous system, and any attempt to breathe consciously in a manner which threatens survival (for instance, holding the breath beyond one's capacity) is overridden by this regulatory system. Responses to many emotions are also involuntary. The symptoms of acute anxiety, the "blush" of embarrassment, and a trembling fit of rage are expressed directly by the autonomic nervous system, often bypassing conscious control. We can all identify how we characteristically respond to specific emotions time after time. That we have these reactions in common with the experiences of most other people indicates a common fundamental psychophysiological response.

Paradoxical breathing is seen in conjunction with a sudden shock or surprise. One reflexively gasps when startled, expanding the chest while tensing the abdomen. If a situation which elicits paradoxical breathing occurs frequently, either because of the presence of much stimulation from the environment or because of an excessive sensitivity to environmental cues, the body will accommodate itself to this mode of functioning, gradually offering less and less resistance to it. Then, after being accustomed to this abnormal pattern, the body risks becoming less specific in its application of this pattern. Relatively minor stresses may then also begin to initiate the same response. And if, as has been previously suggested, breathing itself is intimately associated with the original emotional atmosphere and can in turn reinforce or recreate it, a vicious cycle ensues. Breathing therapy then becomes much more complicated than simply dealing with a set of muscular movements. It becomes a potential tool for intervention in interrupting or controlling undesired emotional response patterns.

Another way to look at breathing is to observe the quality of breath flow. Is it smooth and continuous or is it irregular and choppy? Based upon one's own experiences, one can see that emotions can profoundly affect this flow. Sorrow, pain, and anger, for instance, each disrupt the smooth, relaxed pattern. As with other types of breathing, irregularities in flow also tell something of the state of the physical body. This is especially true of apneic disturbances, or interruptions in the flow of breath. These breathing pauses can occur at various points in the cycle of inhalation/exhalation, varying in duration from a fraction of a second to a minute, and occurring during both sleep and wakefulness.

Of the different possible types of breathing pauses, sleep apnea has received much attention in popular and medical circles. In this syndrome, breathing pauses, lasting up to one minute in severe cases, occur throughout sleep. As one would expect, this has definite detrimental effects on health, at least in its extreme forms, for breathing pauses are often accompanied by elevated blood pressure and a decrease in blood oxygen levels. The latter may fall to such low levels, in fact, that one actually turns blue for a few seconds, and in over half of one group of patients studied, the blood pressure remained elevated throughout the day. Various psychological traits were also noted in people with sleep apnea. Anxiety, occasional confusion, depression, and decreased sexual drive, as well as diminished mentation, occurred more frequently in those who had extreme cases of sleep apnea.

This is a fascinating bit of information, but it was thought not to be of much practical value, considering the small number of people with sleep apnea. However, a study examining "normal" hospital staff volunteers found that two thirds of the men had periods of sleep apnea, in association with low blood oxygen levels, lasting longer than ten seconds. Oddly enough, only a very small number of women experienced any apneic periods at all, none of them associated with low oxygen levels.

The high incidence of sleep apnea in men and the disparity between the sexes in this regard has yet to be systematically explored, though some tentative theories exist. For instance, the association of sleep apnea with periods of low blood oxygenation levels and elevated blood pressure suggests that heart functioning may be affected. The heart is composed of several muscular chambers whose function is to propel blood throughout the body. If the blood pressure is elevated, the heart must work harder, using more oxygen to pump the same amount of blood against this increased resistance. If, at the same time, blood oxygen levels fall, as in sleep apnea, this could create a temporary energy shortage for the heart. Repeating this process frequently, every night for years, could conceivably have a cumulative adverse effect on heart functioning. If one then considers that the death rate from heart disease is much higher in men than in women, might the incidence of heart disease and sleep apnea be related? Does sleep apnea causally affect the development of heart disease? Can modification of this breathing type then exert a therapeutic or preventative effect on the development of heart disease?

These questions have yet to be answered. There is, however, some evidence to support the need for further research into the interrelationship between apnea and heart disease. For many years, nasal surgeons have been studying the relationship of nasal function and air movement through the nose in an effort to diagnose and assess the effects of nasal surgery. Different nasal breathing patterns have been described as a by-product of this testing, including an apneic pattern, the "mid-cycle rest." (This was defined, essentially, as a rapid exhalation, followed by a pause lasting anywhere from a fraction of a second to as long as five seconds after each breath.) For several years, based upon extensive clinical experience and some pilot studies, a number of rhinologists have claimed that the mid-cycle rest is associated with an increased incidence of heart disease. It is interesting to note the similarities between the two studies although the relationship needs to be studied more intensively.

In summary, then, whether making manifest the potential energy locked in nutrient food, or influencing the functional state of the cardiovascular system, or altering autonomic nervous system functioning and emotional states, the breath plays a crucial role in maintaining the integrity of the human organism. Breathing is a fundamental physiological activity which touches man's functioning on numerous levels, and as such it is a window through which these levels can be observed and manipulated. The deceptive simplicity of such a seemingly mundane process has resulted in its being overlooked in the past amidst the sophistication and complexity of our technological society. Only recently have we begun to explore some of the grosser aspects of breathing, generating a torrent of questions and speculations in the process. The results of these explorations promise to be of great practical value in understanding and modifying disease processes.

CHAPTER THREE

FOLLOWING YOUR NOSE: NASAL FUNCTION AND ENERGY

Rudolph Ballentine, M.D.

FOR SOME REASON people don't pay much attention to the nose. Except for the cosmetic effects of its shape, it is usually regarded as little more than an opening through which air enters. If that were its sole purpose, however, people might suppose that it would be constructed differently; it should be wide and open. But the nose is actually the narrowest place in the respiratory tract. It is like a bottleneck; it is the one place where the airflow is most constricted as the air goes into the lungs. If you compare the work required to pull the air in and out of the nose, it is 150 percent of what it would be to move the air through the mouth. This is quite a difference, and it exists even when your nose is not stuffed up. When we stop to consider that we breathe eighteen to twenty thousand times a day, we can begin to appreciate the amount of extra work done in twenty-four hours simply to get the air in and out of the nose instead of the mouth. This process uses a great deal of energy, so there must be a good reason for it.

There are several good reasons. The nose does much more than simply let the air in. Medical specialists who have studied diseases of the nose (rhinologists) can list nearly thirty distinct functions that it performs. It filters, moisturizes, directs the airflow, warms the air, registers the sense of smell, brings in oxygen, creates mucus, provides a route of drainage for the sinuses, and affects the nervous system. It has a number of other functions, too, but these are the best understood.

Anatomy and Physiology of the Nose

The word *nose* is actually a somewhat ambiguous term. To the average person it means the protrusion visible on the middle of the face. But to physicians and physiologists it also means a mysterious and complex internal passageway that somehow involves the sinuses and the sense of smell. For this reason it is perhaps more accurate to think of there being two distinct divisions of the nose: the external and the internal. Humans are unique, in terms of the external nose, for animals have no "nose" in this sense. Although animals do have internal passageways, which are often intricate and serve a variety of important purposes, only humans have this peculiar facial protuberance. Other animals have only simple openings, or holes, through which the air enters the internal nasal cavity. Even our closest relative, the ape, doesn't really have a nose. While there are two nostrils, the profile of an ape shows nothing so prominent as the structure we sport. The shape of the external nose, however, plays an important role in preparing air for inhalation. This is why people who originated in different climates have differently shaped noses. A long, big nose that heats the air before it gets inside is characteristic of those who live in cooler climates and also of those who live in climates, such as the Middle East, where the air is very dry. A warm, moist climate, on the other hand, requires much less processing of the air, making the wide, open nostrils of the inhabitants of tropical jungles a recognizable trait.

The external nose also serves to gather air and accelerate its flow, forming a rapid jet that enters the cavity within the face, the internal nose. As we shall see later, the way that the stream of air is aimed inside the head can be of extreme importance. There are two parts to the external nose. One part is bone. If we feel the base of the nose we will find it to be quite hard and rigid. Moving outward, we encounter a softer area. This is made of cartilage. The first little compartment in the external nose is called the vestibule, and it is formed primarily by the two wings, or alae, of the nose which flare out on each side of it. Because they are cartilage, and relatively flexible, they tend to be influenced by gravity, so if we lie on our side the uppermost nostril will tend to be pulled downward and partially close in a valve-like way.

Moving further up the nose, there are a number of small bones and cartilages put together in an intricate way and attached to a series of bones, whose assembly is also complex, at the base of the nose. When the nose is broken, it is essentially the bony parts at the root of the nose that are fractured. The flexible part, however, can also be injured, particularly internally. Inside and toward the tip of the nose, the septum, which divides the external nose into two passageways, is also made of cartilage. Further back it is bony. Either part of it can be damaged, and this may result in the familiar "deviated septum," which tends to close off one nostril and favor the other.

As we move internally, we find that the nasal passageway expands, the dimensions of the internal nose being much larger than the vestibule. The floor of the internal nose happens also to be the roof of the mouth, and is called the palate. If we move our tongue backward, we find a place where the roof of the mouth suddenly becomes softer. This, the soft palate, is made up of soft tissue only without the bony palate involved, and it ends in a little teardrop-shaped organ we call the uvula. Just as the floor of the nose is the roof of the mouth, so is the roof of the nose also the floor of the brain and of the cavities which house the eyeballs. In other words, we are speaking of a three-story structure. The brain, eyes, and optic nerves occupy the top floor, and the mouth occupies the bottom floor. In between, on the middle floor, is the nasal cavity.

That puts the internal nose in an interesting place since anything going on inside of it is closely related to the brain, the nervous system, the pituitary gland (which is located in the floor of the brain), and many other strategic structures. In addition, the first cranial nerve, which is the olfactory nerve responsible for the sense of smell, enters the nasal cavity and has its nerve endings in the uppermost parts of that compartment. This means that in order to smell something, we have to direct the flow of air up toward the top part of the nasal cavity. To do this, we need to create a rather brisk jet of air entering the external nose. In other words, we sniff, and this propels a rapid stream of air inward and upward which reaches the nerve endings of the olfactory nerve.

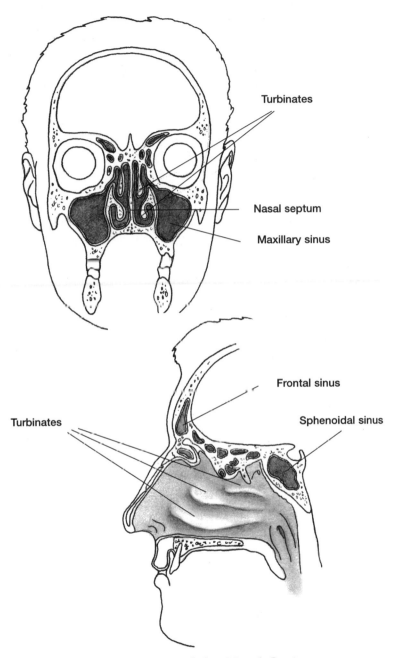

Cross Section of the Nasal Cavity

The shape of the internal nose determines the path that the air follows. What we discover when we look closely inside the nasal cavity is that its walls are far from smooth. It is full of all sorts of strange and convoluted shapes and structures. We might be prompted to conclude that the nose is some kind of junkyard where all sorts of odd organs have been thrown that didn't seem to fit anywhere else. Actually, however, it is all intricately engineered. In fact, to really understand the nose properly, we would have to be well-versed in aerodynamics, for each bend and curve and nook and cranny has its purpose. Everything is cleverly designed to move the air in particular directions.

The most prominent structures filling the nasal cavity are the three seashell-like bulges that we can catch a glimpse of as we look up inside it. These are called the turbinates. As their name implies, their function is to stir and circulate the air as it enters the nose, and the result is that the stream of air passes over a much greater surface than it would otherwise. The turbinates thereby have a marked effect on the moisture content and temperature of the entering air, for as the air enters, it passes over the warm, moist turbinates, picking up humidity and heat. This process prepares the air so that it will not be a shock to the delicate tissues of the lungs.

As the air leaves the lungs, the opposite reaction occurs. As it passes over the turbinates, which have just been cooled and dried by the incoming air, the outgoing air now re-warms and moistens them. In that way the turbinates help prevent the loss of heat and moisture from the body. Some animals, like seals, have large and complex turbinates whose surface area exceeds that of their skin. Since they live on the edge of cold, windy, salt waters, recovery of water and heat from exhaled air must be extremely important for these animals in maintaining their body temperature and conserving a salt-free internal moisture. In humans, whose turbinates are much smaller, this function is apparently less significant. In cold weather, however, the turbinates and external nose are cooled enough so that as people exhale, the moisture in the warm air condenses on these colder structures much as moisture condenses on the cold window of an automobile, and they often develop a characteristic dripping. In fact, in very cold weather it is not uncommon to have an icicle form on the tip of the nose.

The turbinates serve, then, to baffle the air, to stir it up, and to create a certain amount of turbulence. Too much turbulence, however, may cause difficulty in breathing, for it may become a great effort to pull air through such a tortuous course (the degree of turbulence depends more on the arrangement of the turbinates and other structures than on the actual size of the passageway). Thus it is that some people have difficulty breathing even though they have extremely large nasal passages.

The Mucus Blanket

As the turbulent air is brought more thoroughly into contact with the surface of the turbinates and nasal lining, it results in a more effective deposition of dust and other particles. To cope with this problem, the inside of the nose is lined with a covering called a mucous membrane, so-named because it has the special property of being able to secrete mucus. Though nasal mucus is more often than not considered to be a nuisance, it actually performs a vital function, for it picks up dust and debris and carries it out of the nose.

This includes not only particles, but microbes such as bacteria, viruses, fungi, and whatever else might be floating about in the air that can invade the delicate tissues of the nose and cause an infection. So the mucus cannot be allowed to build up, dry out, and accumulate. Some provision must be made for its removal, and the system facilitating this process is ingenious and fascinating. Since we cannot simply lift out the nasal air filter and replace it every five thousand miles, there must be some self-cleaning mechanism in the nose. The mucus accomplishes this by constantly moving. Obviously, gravity is not the sole cause of this movement. Otherwise our nose would always be dripping, and normally the mucus does not run out of our nostrils. In fact, mucus often moves against gravity, moving upward and backward, across the nasal cavity walls and toward the throat, where it is swallowed and enters the esophagus. This thin coating of mucus is continuously in motion, and the result is a sort of "mucus blanket" which moves along, carrying everything with it.

The mysterious movement of this blanket is due to millions of tiny hair-like structures which grow out of the mucous membrane. Called cilia, their untiring, consistent, and continual motion is one of the miraculous phenomena of biology. That tiny subcellular structures, driven by a simple mechanism, can move without rest twenty-four hours a day is no mean feat, to say the least. Moreover, their movement is coordinated; each of them works in concert with the others. Because there are so many of them, the blanket of mucus is passed over the cilia like someone handed arm-over-arm above the heads of a crowd. Thus the mucus blanket is continuously in motion, and as a result, any microbes caught in the mucus blanket are kept moving fast enough so they never have an opportunity to escape or settle in. Eventually this mucus ends up in the intestinal tract, where the digestive enzymes dissolve both it and the microbes it carries.

This is a beautiful system as long as it works properly. Unfortunately, sometimes it fails. What makes it break down? If the mucus is too viscous or thick, then it easily dries out and adheres to the cilia and mucous membrane, and at that point crusts will build up and microbes begin to invade. This is often the beginning of a cold.

The opposite extreme can also be problematic. If the mucus is too liquid, too runny, then it drips down around the cilia, and they can't hold it together and move it as an intact coating or continuous "blanket." The result is the development of a watery nasal drip. Again, the mucus blanket has become ineffective in protecting against infection, and when it is in this condition, inflammation can easily begin. This is a frequent component of hay fever. For such reasons the consistency of the mucus is important; as long as it is of the correct composition and viscosity, everything generally functions well.

One of the primary factors determining the composition of mucus is diet. Too much starchy food as well as milk products, for instance, are notorious for creating a thicker and more viscous mucus. In the East this is explained by defining mucus not only as a secretion, but also as an excretion. A secretion is something manufactured by the body to serve a definite purpose that is constructive; an excretion, by contrast, is something of which we are ridding ourselves. Normally, mucus is primarily a secretion. It becomes an excretion when some other excretory function of the body is not performing up to par. That is to say, mucus becomes an excretion when the lungs, skin, bowels, kidneys, and menses are unable to rid the body of wastes that have accumulated, and mucus production increases and begins to take over some of this function.

Constipation is common in our culture. We often use antiperspirants to prevent the skin from taking its share of the excretory load. Even our breathing, which, when properly regulated, can help rid the body of certain volatile wastes, is often shallow and fails to serve this purpose. To make the situation worse, since our diet often includes many processed (and therefore injured and damaged) foods, we have more of a load of wastes to get rid of in the first place, and with many of our excretory channels obstructed, we are often desperate to unload from the body an accumulation of useless material. The result is often only offensive body odor or bad breath, but eventually a crisis may be reached, and the body seizes the opportunity to discharge quantities of mucus. This is the familiar "cold" that comes on the heels of overeating, a bad diet, or constipation. (In another era, grandmother was quick to recommend a laxative at the first signs of a cold in order to prevent its developing into something severe.)

Normally the mucus and mucous membranes function in a neat, tidy, and orderly way. But when we force them to do so, they become accessory routes of excretion. Then the composition of the mucus is no longer determined by what is ideal in terms of its protective function. Rather, it is determined by what needs to be thrown off, and it becomes either too liquid, or too thick, or otherwise abnormal. The result is not only the discharge of quantities of mucus, but also the absence of effective protection by the mucous membranes, with subsequent irritation, inflammation, and often infection. Fortunately, such infection is seldom severe; it is

apparently regarded by the body as a lesser evil than the retention of large quantities of useless and encumbering
wastes.

This explanation helps us understand why dry air is sometimes so troublesome. If the mucus is already too much on
the thick side, then a bit of dry air will immediately cause
caking and the accumulation of crusts of mucus in the nose,
which in turn cause discomfort and irritation. This is especially true in areas where a jet of air strikes continuously. Because of the structure of the internal nose, there are certain
areas where this is more likely to happen. For instance, the
inflowing jet of air is deflected against the back of the nasal
cavity and moves downward, striking a point at the back of
the throat. Here, the air is particularly likely to deposit debris, dust, and microbes, so the body has responded by sta-
tioning there a powerful concentration of lymphoid tissue
which is capable of mustering white blood cells and anti-
bodies to fight any threatening invaders. This accumulation
of lymphoid tissues, though, sometimes becomes quite large
and can obstruct the throat. Surgical removal of the tonsil,
as the structure is called, to prevent this problem used to be
quite common. It took years for physicians to realize that
some purposeful and valuable tissue was lost in the process,
and the operation of tonsillectomy became progressively un-
popular.

Another frequent problem in the area of the nasal cavity
is sinusitis. The sinuses are cavities in the facial structure that
adjoin and open into the nasal cavity (see diagram on page
49). The largest sinuses are located above each eye and in
each cheekbone. Lined with mucous membrane, the sinuses
can also secrete mucus, but they should, of course, remain
hollow. Though their function is not fully understood, we

know that in part they lend resonance to the voice by vibrating with the vocal cords. Besides the two main parts of sinuses, there are others deeper in the head, behind the nose, up under the brain, and behind the eyes. These are smaller than the main sinuses, however, and less likely to cause trouble, though sometimes they can also become painful and inflamed.

Tiny passageways lead from each sinus down into the nasal cavity, and it is through these tiny passageways that the sinuses are able to drain and rid themselves of their own mucus blanket. Inflammation and problems in the sinuses result when one of the tiny passageways becomes obstructed, or clogged up, and the sinus cannot maintain a free circulation of air and mucus between itself and the nasal cavity. Normally, air moves in and out of the sinus as the stream of air flows through the nasal cavity, but when the passageway from the sinus into the nose becomes obstructed, this airflow stops, and the mucous membranes lining the sinus begin to absorb the air. This creates a kind of partial vacuum inside the sinus, and the result is to pull not only mucus, but even blood and tissue fluids, into the sinus, creating a severe irritation, pressure, and pain. What follows is what we call sinusitis and sometimes sinus headache.

The little passageways leading from the sinuses into the nasal cavity generally enter underneath the turbinates, and when these areas collect mucus that is dried or crusted, it may obstruct the passageways to the sinuses and provoke such sinus problems. One way to prevent and gradually eliminate these problems is the systematic use of a technique called *neti* (the nasal wash). This involves pouring a warm, mildly salty solution of water into one nostril and allowing it to flow out of the other. This dissolves and washes away mucus and allows the mucous membrane to function properly again. It also often frees the openings of the passageways through which the sinuses drain. Many people recoil at the idea of pouring water into the nose, but detailed studies of nasal function reveal that this is far from an unnatural procedure. Actually, it is natural to have salt water inside the nose since it is not only the sinuses which empty into the internal nose, but the lachrymal duct as well.

Tears, which are salty, are produced by the lachrymal glands under the upper eyelid. They course down across the surface of the eye, keeping it moist, and are picked up by a tiny duct in the inner, lower corner of the eye. The tears are then carried by this duct into the nasal passage, where they drain along with the sinuses. When one weeps and produces large amounts of tears, the nose begins to "run," prompting that person, in the midst of an emotional scene, to reach for a handkerchief. Even without emotion, however, tears are constantly flowing across the eye (though in smaller quantities) and constantly entering the little tunnel which carries them to the inside of the nose. In other words, a continuous input of salty water into the nose occurs at all times. Salt water is, in fact, the natural "wash" for the linings of the nasal cavity.

To capitalize on this fact, the nasal wash should be done with water that is of the same composition as tears. It should be exactly that salty, and it should be at body temperature. When done this way, the nasal wash is soothing and does not irritate the lining of the nose. Iodized salt and chlorinated or chemicalized water are unnatural and may be irritating.

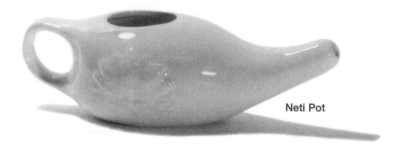

Neti Pot

Nasal Wash Instructions

Regular use of a Neti Pot cleanses and restores health to the internal sinus passages. In yoga, breathing freely through both nostrils is also said to aid in harmonizing the active and passive systems of the body, and so the neti wash has been found to be a helpful practice before meditation.

Mix well a heaping one-quarter teaspoon of finely ground salt, such as table salt (use a slightly rounded one-half teaspoon with coarse varieties, like kosher salt) and lukewarm water in your Neti Pot. (The amount of salt may vary slightly with each person.) Make sure the salt is completely dissolved before using the solution. Bring the spout to the nose and bend forward over the sink, with the head tilted to the side and slightly forward. As the water flows through the upper nostril, make slight adjustments with your head and the Neti Pot, if necessary, to allow the water to flow out of the other nostril.

After the pot empties, blow freely into the sink through both nostrils to clear the nose of excess water and mucus. Do not close off one nostril when doing this because it could force the water back into the ear. If there are any further problems in clearing the nostrils, kneel down and bring your forehead to the floor so that your hips are above the level of the head. Blow freely through the nostrils as before. Turning the head to either side while doing so could aid this process as well. After completing the neti wash through the nostrils in one direction, repeat the same steps on the opposite side.

After some proficiency is gained in this method, one may also learn to direct the water from the nose out through the mouth, again by making slight adjustments with the position of the head and the Neti Pot, and using the back of the mouth to draw the water in for spitting it out. This method is also helpful for cleansing and ridding the nasal passages of excess mucus and dirt, and restoring health to the sinus membranes.

A mucous membrane also lines the passageways that carry air down into the lungs and chest, for the bronchi are fitted with the same kind of lining as the nose, which secretes mucus to keep the passages moist. Otherwise the air would dry and injure them. The mucus secreted in these passageways is moved upward by the cilia, all the way to the throat, day and night. During the day the cilia ordinarily have to work against gravity, but at night, when one lies down, their work is easier since they don't have to push the mucus uphill. For this reason, at night a great deal more mucus comes up to the throat, is cleared, and swallowed. That process goes on without ceasing.

Normally, the mucus entering the gastrointestinal tract is dissolved by the juices which also kill all the microbes. This is a sort of internal ecological system in which mucus is broken down and recycled, and which prevents a variety of problems. However, problems will develop as soon as mucus is excessive or when digestive juices are not present. Unfortunately, the intestinal tract tends to quiet down and rest during the night; because digestion is a process that is not normally active at this time, less digestive juice is secreted. Therefore, if the mucus is excessive, a stomach full of it can accumulate by morning. For this reason many people wake up feeling quite uncomfortable until they eat something, which serves to either dilute the mucus or push it out of the stomach. This is especially true of people with such problems as lung diseases, emphysema, and asthma, who tend to produce a great deal of mucus.

For such persons, a morning wash is often recommended. Here, a large quantity of saline solution is swallowed, and then thrown up. This brings out the mucus from the stomach—a simple but sound hygienic principle. The technique is called *gaj karni* (the upper wash), and most well-trained yoga instructors are able to instruct others in its use. (This technique is performed on an empty stomach. Inducing vomiting to empty the stomach contents after a meal, in order to prevent weight gain, is an extremely unhealthy practice.)

Smokers, especially, tend to develop a great deal of mucus. A lot of this is mobilized and thrown out if they stop smoking, and after this cleansing period the lungs begin to recover. The accumulation of mucus in smokers (which creates their characteristic rattling cough and their inability to bring out the mucus that accumulates) is due to both the irritation caused by smoke and coal tar, and to the destruction of cilia. The contents of cigarette smoke totally decimate the cilia in the mucous membranes, and this means that there is no mechanism for bringing the mucus back up out of the lungs to the throat. So it accumulates. After one stops smoking the cilia gradually begin to regenerate and to handle the mucus normally again.

Laterality

If we return to the nose for a moment and reexamine its lining, we discover that underneath the mucous membrane layer is another, much thicker, layer of tissue that is spongy and can fill with large quantities of blood. This is called "erectile" tissue, and it is found only in a few areas of the body: the genitals, the breasts, and the lining of the nose. Within this tissue are tiny microscopic passageways that receive blood, causing the tissue to expand, and this engorgement is the basis of erection in the penis and the clitoris. There is a close relationship between these organs and the lining of the nose. In fact, this is the basis of a syndrome, familiar to ear, nose, and throat doctors, which often occurs with newly-married couples. Just after marriage, during a period of continual sexual stimulation, the lining of the nose becomes chronically engorged and clogged up through a sympathetic kind of interaction. This is called "honeymoon nose."

Sigmund Freud, in his pioneering work with sexuality, was very conscious of the interaction between the sexual organs and the nose. In fact, he originally developed his basic psychoanalytic theory through his correspondence with Wilhelm Fliess, an ear, nose, and throat specialist. The interest which drew them together was the reflexes that exist between the nasal lining and the reproductive organs. One of Freud's earliest theories, developed in conjunction with Fliess, was that there is a "nasal reflex neurosis." Though he later lost interest in this phenomenon, other physicians went on to elaborate on the research and to discover many interesting interrelationships. It was found, for example, that menstrual cramps were often related to an inflammation and discoloration of certain specific areas in the lining of the nose. When these were anesthetized with a small amount of topical anesthetic, the menstrual pains would disappear. For some time in Germany, as a matter of fact, menstrual pain was effectively treated through cauterization, or permanent destruction, of the nerve endings in selected regions of the nasal lining.

The swelling and shrinking of the nasal erectile tissue does more, however, than simply warm the air and reflect sexual overstimulation. In fact, there is a constant, regular, and predictable pattern of swelling and shrinkage that the lining of the nose follows which is closely related to the whole concept of laterality in human physiology.

For instance, as the tissue covering the turbinates and the septum within one nostril swell, the tissues on the opposite side tend to become less swollen. As a result, one nostril gradually and increasingly becomes obstructed so that the flow of air is shifted to the other side. Consequently, there is a right-left dimension of breath flow: it can flow either predominantly through the right nostril or predominantly through the left nostril. If nothing is done to interfere with the rhythmic functioning of the body, this will tend to alternate in a predictable fashion. The breath will be flowing predominantly through one nostril for about an hour and forty-five minutes to two hours, after which it becomes predominant in the other side, for flow increases in one side until it reaches a peak, and then it begins to decrease. Soon thereafter, most of the air begins to flow through the opposite nostril.

Though this is apparently a natural biological rhythm, it can be interfered with by emotional disturbance, irregular schedules of meals or sleep, and irritation in the nose due to pollution, infection, and other disrupting forces. If, however, one is healthy, tranquil, and calm, and living in a sensible, regular way, then the alternation of the airflow between one nostril and another follows a definite regular rhythm. This has been well-documented in research laboratories both in the West and in the East. Today, this is technically called an "infradian rhythm," but its recognition is hardly a recent advance of science. In fact, it was described in great detail by the ancient yogis who, as a result of cultivating techniques of self-observation to a high degree, were able to perceive and catalog such subtle changes in the body.

Moreover, the *svara* yogis, adepts who focused on the science of breath, made intricate correlations between the way the breath was flowing and various psychological and physiological states. They observed, for example, that having the right or left nostril open would gear us toward one activity or another in the world. If individuals breathe through the right side, they said, they tend to become more active and aggressive, more alert and more oriented toward the external world. Breathing through the left side, on the other hand, produces a quieter, more passive psychological state, one more oriented toward the inner world. This is all reminiscent of what has been written recently on right brain/left brain, and it seems logical to ask whether right-nostril flow is correlated with the predominance of one hemisphere over another. In fact, research work is in progress to answer this question.

The distinction between right- and left-nostril breathing, however, is more than psychological. It is said that the flow of air through the right nostril gears the internal organs toward more active physiological processes too, processes such as digesting food, for example. Therefore, students of svara yoga were careful to open the right nostril before eating.

Drinking water, by contrast, is a more passive kind of intake, and fluids were customarily taken with the left nostril open. Since they considered the side through which the air was flowing to be extremely important, the breath was attuned properly before any particular activity was undertaken. This was thought to gear both the body and the mind, preparing one mentally, emotionally, and physiologically for a particular activity.

The science of breath was well-known to the ancient people of India. They practiced it consistently and as a matter of course. Today, however, since most people have not developed an awareness of breath, the practices currently taught as a part of yoga are designed to help one become more sensitive to and conscious of the flow of air and what it is doing at any given moment. Such breathing exercises can also help one restore regularity, rhythm, and balance to nostril alternation.

The most commonly used of these yoga breathing exercises is called *nadi shodhanam* (alternate nostril breathing), a technique in which one deliberately changes the flow of air from one side to the other, regularly and rhythmically, through exerting pressure on the valve or lateral wall of one nostril or the other. To perform this properly, diaphragmatic breathing should have already been mastered so that the flow of air is smooth, even, consistent, and well-regulated.

Nadi Shodhanam

To begin this technique, sit straight as though for meditation, in whatever position is comfortable, but with the head, neck, and trunk relatively erect. Usually the thumb of the right hand is used to close off the right nostril while the

ring finger of the same hand is used to close off the left nostril. If you find it helpful, you can brace the hand by placing the index and middle fingers on the bridge of the nose
between the eyes (if you don't find that to be a distraction).

First, exhale through the active nostril—the one that is
most open. Then inhale through the same nostril. At the
end of the inhalation, close off that nostril with the finger,
allowing the exhalation to begin on the other side. At the
end of that exhalation, inhale through the same nostril, thus
starting the process again. Repeat this alternation three
times so that you breathe a complete cycle through each
nostril three times, for a total of six breaths. This is ordinarily called a "round." It is customary to perform a second
and then a third such round so that you complete a total of
nine inhalations and nine exhalations through each nostril.
Between rounds, you ordinarily take three breaths through
both nostrils.

In doing the exercise, you should remember two things:
to breathe slowly and gently, but not so slowly that it is a
strain or that you run out of breath; and to breathe silently.
If the breath is allowed to flow gently and smoothly, then
less turbulence is created, and no sound vibration should result. To accomplish these two goals, you must concentrate
completely on the breathing itself. If the mind is allowed to
wander to other subjects during the process, the breathing
will become irregular, jerky, noisy, or otherwise disruptive.
It is also important to remain relaxed and calm during the
exercise.

This is only one of three variants. The second (which is
explained in chapter four) involves exhalation through one
side with inhalation through the other, and the third involves three complete cycles through one nostril before

changing to the other side. Some students choose to do one variant for the full three rounds, while other people do a round of each variant. Consistency is probably helpful, and the variant described in the text is quite suitable for the beginner to use exclusively.

Practicing this technique enables people to appreciate the difference between the experience of breathing through one side and breathing through the other, and they also increase their awareness of the nature of laterality. Nadi shodhanam is a study rather than simply a mechanical exercise. It is both educational and coordinating. It brings a dimension of existence which has been forgotten back into awareness, and it helps to restore coordination between the two sides of the body. We would be most embarrassed to admit that we didn't appreciate the difference between lifting the left arm and the right arm, but most people, when asked, cannot say which nostril they're breathing through at the moment. If it is true that the right side activates a whole set of psychological and physiological functions and the left side brings into play a different set, then it would certainly be valuable to have access to an awareness of which nostril is flowing at any given moment.

The importance of this awareness becomes especially obvious when we discover techniques which enable us to change voluntarily the flow of air from one side to the other. For example, if I lie on my left side, then the right nostril will open. It was long thought that this was because gravity pulled the blood into the lower nostril, engorging the lining, causing the turbinates to swell, and closing off the "down" side. More recently, research has demonstrated that it is not actually gravity which is responsible for this shift; rather, it is the pressure exerted between the down arm and the side of the chest on which one is lying. This apparently sets up a reflex which automatically dilates the nostril that is higher and closes off the one which is lower, on the side where the pressure is. In any case, if I stay on one side for awhile, the opposite nostril will open. It is for this reason that the yoga manuals recommend that one lie on the left side after meals, opening the right nostril and stimulating the digestive process. Traditionally, too, it is said that when individuals go to bed, they should lie on the left side for five or ten minutes, activating the right nostril to create increased body heat. As soon as they are warm and comfortable, they should turn to the right, allowing the left nostril to open. Doing so relaxes, calms, and prepares them for sleep.

While a rhythmic alternation of airflow between one side and the other is considered natural and healthy, the persistent closure of one nostril and flow of air through the other for more than a few hours is thought to be a harbinger of disease. If the breath stays in one side for six or eight hours, some illness is thought to be on its way, and if the condition lasts for a day or more, the situation is said to be grave. The breath is thought to be related to the *prana* (flow of energy) in the subtle psychophysiological totality, the imbalances of which are seen as preceding the outward manifestation of disease.

Shaping the Air Currents

While we have discussed and looked at the structure and shape of the nose and nasal cavity, there is another aspect of breathing which also has its own shape and structure. That is the air current itself. The pathways through which it flows—the currents and eddies and crosscurrents—all make up an incredibly complex and intricate pattern of airflow that will vary from person to person, depending upon each person's nasal cavity and external nose. Just as the banks of a river shape the flow of the water, so does the nasal cavity and upper respiratory passage shape and direct the flow of air. According to the ancient yogis, this was an extremely critical issue, the flow of air being related to the flow of energy, or prana, and the patterns according to which it energized the body and mind.

While these yogic concepts have not been thoroughly investigated by modern research techniques, it is certainly true that many rhinologists agree on the importance of the shape of the nose. Here they differ from plastic surgeons who are concerned with cosmetic effects. Their work, rather, is primarily directed toward improved functioning of the nose— that is, altering its internal structure so that misshapen passageways are restored and the airflow is corrected. Some rhinologists feel that this has an incredible impact both on the psychology and physiology of the person concerned. There are documented cases, for instance, in which the internal distortion of the nose and the abnormal flow of air so affected the people that they became mentally unbalanced. On the other hand, there are documented cases in which psychological disorders developed after nasal surgery. It is not uncommon for individuals to notice, after extensive restructuring of the inner nose through surgery, that they feel different.

The yogis would not be surprised by this, feeling strongly that the shape of the inner passageways and the shape of the flow of air that results is an important factor in molding both mental states and personality. According to the Eastern way of thinking, this movement of airflow affects the way in which prana is supplied to the body and brain, and in this way it influences both emotions and mind. Prana is said to nourish the conscious mind and make it flow, pushing it in one direction or another.

This perspective on breathing has remained foreign to Western science. Nevertheless, nose surgeons who are skilled and accomplished work with this variable, intuitively structuring and reshaping the inner nose with sensitive and experienced hands. Such surgery is a crucial undertaking and not one to be taken lightly, for if the ancient ideas about breath are even partially true, to have the nose changed is to tamper with a very formative part of oneself. It should be done by an extremely competent and experienced person. Even setting a broken nose can be a delicate matter, and certainly nose surgery which ignores functional effects can be a disaster. A recent case (seen by the author) of a man who had had his turbinates removed because they seemed to obstruct his nasal passage illustrates this point. Postoperatively, the patient was so completely mentally confused that he found it necessary to give up his profession.

Of course, the primary domain of rhinologists, or nose surgeons, is the bony structure that underlies the shape of the nasal cavity. In order to determine whether surgery is required, rhinologists shrink all of the erectile tissue lining the nasal cavity with sprays and topical applications, and then they do tests for airflow. If flow can be restored to normal through this technique, they assume that no surgery is needed.

Actually, it is rare that the bony structure itself plays such a large role in shaping the air. It is rather the engorgement of the spongy erectile tissue which changes, shifts, and causes the pattern of airflow to alter. As we have seen, the turbinates on one side engorge, closing off that nostril and resulting in a switch of airflow to the other side. This is not so simple as a matter of right or left, however. On each side there are three large turbinates as well as the inner surface of the septum, each of which is covered with erectile tissue. The degree and location of swelling in each of these can vary, and the permutations and combinations are incredible. The result is a complex, continually changing pattern of airflow which can only be likened to the result of driving a large, heavy-duty vehicle with three separate gearshifts, each gearshift having a number of positions, so that the resulting combinations are numerous.

From the perspective of ancient Eastern ideas about breathing, the turbinates, by combining in various ways to create a varying pattern of airflow, help gear us to different activities. This is a continuously changing phenomenon, both influencing and resulting from emotional and mental states as well as physiological functions. The pattern of engorgement in the turbinates and the resulting shape of airflow resemble a central clearinghouse or switchboard, where all the body's functions are having an effect, and are in turn being affected. In fact, research has shown that the flow of air touching the surface of various areas of the turbinates triggers neuronal responses that set up reflexes throughout the body. In other words, a specific current of air sends out ripples into both the lungs and the nervous system that affect the whole person. In the ancient scriptures specific descriptions are given of various patterns of airflow and their relationship to personality states and physiological function. Laboratory research is gradually gaining the sophisticated technology needed to be able to look into and disprove or verify these ancient ideas.

Nasal Functioning and the Limbic System

Neurophysiologists have found that inhalation not only stimulates the olfactory nerve when the air contains substances that can be sensed with the sense of smell, but it also triggers neuronal messages in the olfactory nerve even when the air is clean. Why this occurs is not known. It is known, however, that the olfactory nerve and the part of the brain that it reaches are integrally connected to the limbic system, that part of the central nervous system which subserves emotional states. We all know that odors are closely connected to emotions, a fact which is put into practice every time a bit of perfume is dabbed behind the ears. To discover, however, that the same brain structures may be brought into play simply through the movement of air is intriguing.

The breath has, then, a profound effect on man's physical and psychological functioning since it is the link between the body and mind. The nose, therefore, as the major portal of breath into the body, plays a crucial role. It prepares and modifies the breath for assimilation by the body, interacting with both the external and internal environment, changing its activity to meet the body's energy demands from moment to moment. An awareness of the functioning of the nose lends an added dimension to both psychological and physiological self-awareness.

CHAPTER FOUR

PORTAL TO HIGHER AWARENESS: THE SCIENCE OF BREATH

Swami Rama

THE SANSKRIT WORD *pranayama* is usually translated as "the science of breath," but this is a limited interpretation. Pranayama literally means "the *ayama* (expansion or manifestation) of *prana* (*pra:* first unit; *na:* energy). Prana is the vital energy of the universe. According to one of the schools of Indian philosophy, the whole universe was projected out of *akasha* (space) through the energy of prana. Akasha is the infinite, all-encompassing material of the universe, and prana is the infinite, all-pervading energy of the universe—cosmic energy. All the diverse forms of this universe are sustained by it. Pranayama is the science which imparts knowledge related to the control of prana. One who has learned to control prana has learned to control all the energies of this universe—physical and mental. He has also learned to control his body and mind.

The mind stands like a wall between us and reality. When the student comes in touch with the finer forces called prana he can learn to control his mind, for it is tightly fastened to prana like a kite to a string. When the string is held skillfully, the kite, which wants to fly here and there, is controlled and flies in the direction desired. All yogic breathing exercises, advanced or basic, enable the student to control his mind by understanding prana. Thus, the science of breath helps the student to bring prana under control in order to attain the higher rungs of spirituality. He who has controlled his breath and prana has also controlled his mind. He who has controlled his mind has also controlled his breath.

All aspects and principles that constitute the universe, or macrocosm, are embodied in all the microcosmic forms that constitute the universe, just as the mighty ocean is completely represented in a single, small drop of water from that ocean. The human body is sustained by the same prana that sustains the universe, and it is through the manifestation of prana that all body functions are possible and coordinated.

According to the ancient manuals of yoga, the cosmic force of prana in the human body is recognized and subdivided on the basis of the ten functions it performs. Of the ten pranas, there are five major and five minor ones. The major pranas are *udana, prana, samana, apana,* and *vyana.* Although the word *prana* is applied to all ten pranas, one of the five major pranas has also been given the name prana for reasons which will soon become clear.

Udana rules the region of the body above the larynx and governs the use of our special senses. Prana rules the region between the larynx and the base of the heart. It governs speech and the vocal apparatus as well as the respiratory system and the muscles associated with it. Samana rules the region between the heart and the navel and governs all the metabolic activity involved in digestion. Apana has its abode below the navel and governs the functions of the kidneys, colon, rectum, bladder, and genitals. Vyana pervades the whole body and governs the relaxation and contraction of all muscles, voluntary and involuntary, as well as the movement of the joints and the structures around them.

The energy of prana is subtle in form. Its most external manifestation is the breath, and of the five major pranas in the human body, prana is the energy that governs the breath. It is through the control of respiration that the yogi proceeds to control the other subtle energies of prana, which may explain the use of the same word for the universal energy as well as for the specific prana governing respiration. The importance of this specific prana in allowing us access to the subtler energies of the cosmic prana is also seen in the fact that what we call death results from the cessation of respiration.

The sequence in which one proceeds from control of the breath to control of the cosmic energy is clearly illustrated in the following story that Swami Vivekananda tells in his book on raja yoga.

There once was a king's minister who fell into disgrace and was imprisoned at the top of a tall tower. The minister asked his faithful wife to come to the tower when darkness had fallen, and to bring with her a long rope, some stout twine, string, silken thread, a beetle, and some honey. Though bewildered by this strange request, the good wife did as he bade her. The minister then asked his wife to tie the silken thread to the beetle, to smear some honey on its horns, and then to set it on the tower wall with its head pointed toward the top of the tower. The beetle, enticed onward by the sweet smell of the honey, slowly made its way to the top of the tower, pulling the silken thread behind it. The minister took hold of the silken thread and then asked his wife to tie the string to the other end of the silken thread. Using the silken thread, he drew up the string. In like manner, he used the string to draw up the stout twine, and the twine to draw up the rope. Then he descended to freedom, using the rope.

In our body the breath is like the silken thread, enabling us to skillfully grasp the string of the nerve impulses; from this we grasp the stout twine of our thoughts, and finally we grasp the rope of prana, thus gaining our ultimate freedom.

Pranayama and the Nervous System

In order to understand the science of pranayama it is necessary to consider the nature and function of the nervous system, for this system coordinates the functions of all the other systems in the body. It is subdivided into the central and the autonomic nervous systems. The central nervous system consists of the brain, twelve pairs of cranial nerves, the spinal cord and thirty-one pairs of spinal nerves. The cranial and spinal nerves spread throughout the body, forming a network of nerve fibers. Efferent, or motor nerve fibers, carry nerve impulses from the brain and spinal cord outward to the nerve endings, and afferent, or sensory nerve fibers, carry nerve impulses from the nerve endings inward to the brain and spinal cord.

To illustrate the functions of the afferent and efferent fibers, consider the case of stubbing your toe. The nerve endings at the toe send nerve impulses along the afferent fibers to the spinal cord and brain. The brain interprets these impulses as pain and reacts by sending motor impulses along the efferent fibers outward to the hands, enabling them to reach out and soothe the injured toe.

Patanjali, the sage who codified yoga science around 200 B.C., explains that the control of prana is the regulation of inhalation and exhalation. This is accomplished by eliminating the pause between inhalation and exhalation, or by expanding the pause through retention. Then, by regulating the motion of the lungs, the heart and the vagus nerve are controlled. The autonomic nervous system regulates processes in our body which are not normally under our voluntary control, such as secretion by the digestive organs, the beating of the heart, and the movement of the lungs. The science of pranayama is thus intimately connected with the autonomic nervous system and brings its functions under conscious control through the functioning of the lungs. Though the act of respiration is for the most part involuntary, voluntary control in this area is easily achieved, for the depth, duration, and frequency of respiration can be consciously modulated quite readily. It is for this reason that control of the breath constitutes an obvious starting point toward attainment of control over the functioning of the autonomic nervous system.

The autonomic nervous system is subdivided into the sympathetic and the parasympathetic systems. As these names indicate, these two subsystems work in seeming opposition to each other, yet the net result is harmonious regulation. The parasympathetic system, for instance, slows down the heart while the sympathetic system accelerates it, and between these two opposing actions the heart rate is regulated. The sympathetic nervous system consists mainly of two vertical rows of ganglia, or nerve cell clusters, arranged on either side of the spinal column. Branches from these gangliated cords spread out to different glands and viscera in the thorax and abdomen, forming integrated

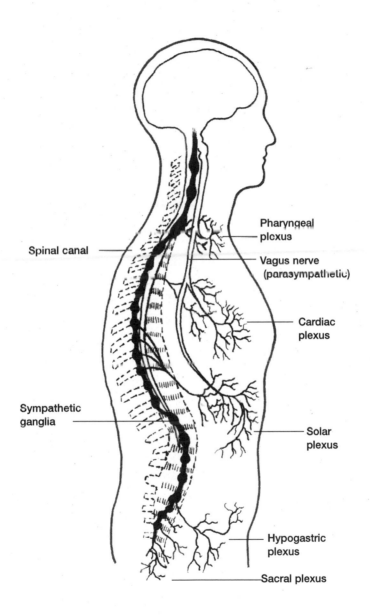

Spinal canal

Pharyngeal plexus

Vagus nerve (parasympathetic)

Cardiac plexus

Sympathetic ganglia

Solar plexus

Hypogastric plexus

Sacral plexus

Autonomic Nervous System

plexuses with nerve branches of the parasympathetic system. The main part of this system is the tenth cranial nerve, also called the vagus, or "wandering," nerve which is connected with the hindbrain and travels downward along the spinal cord through the neck, chest, and abdomen, sending out branches to form various plexuses with the sympathetic system. It ends in a plexus which is connected to the solar plexus, but is also connected with the lower plexuses through filaments.

There are only two known ways of gaining conscious control over the involuntary nervous system. One is by systematically practicing breathing exercises and preparing oneself for understanding the various vehicles and channels of prana. But first the student should learn to regulate the motion of the lungs so that heart function is regulated. Then the right vagus nerve is brought under conscious control, and the portion of the mind that coordinates with the involuntary system becomes accessible to him. There is no such thing as an involuntary system if the student learns to regulate the motion of the lungs. For by doing so, a vast portion of that system is brought under his voluntary control.

The other way of gaining control over the autonomic nervous system is through willpower. The more the mind is dissipated, the more the will is scattered. When the mind is made one-pointed, the willpower is strengthened, and with the help of the willpower the autonomic nervous system functions the way we want it to.

Modern scientists give importance to breathing exercises only from the viewpoint of oxygen intake. Their concern is with the absorption of oxygen in large enough quantities to vitalize the nervous system. But in the science of breath, this is a minor consideration. More detailed knowledge and experience is needed to study the finer forces of life than the mere intake of oxygen and output of carbon dioxide. The ancient manuals of yoga anatomy, for instance, describe a network of several thousand nadis (subtle channels) through which the currents of prana flow, energizing and sustaining all parts of the body as well as the several thousand nadis.

According to some manuals the number of nadis is 72,000 (others mention 350,000). Fourteen are more important than the others, but the most important among these are six: *ida, pingala, sushumna, brahmani, chitrani,* and *vijnani.* Among these six, three are the most important: pingala *(surya),* which flows through the right nostril; ida *(chandra),* which flows through the left nostril; and sushumna, which is a moment when both nostrils flow freely without any obstruction. Expansion of that moment is called *sandhya.* For meditation, the application of sushumna is of prime importance, for after applying sushumna, the meditator cannot be disturbed by noise or other disturbances from the external world, nor by the bubbles of thought arising from the unconscious during meditation.

All three of the major nadis originate at the base of the spine and travel upward. The sushumna nadi is centrally located and travels along the spinal canal. At the level of the larynx it divides into an anterior and a posterior portion, both of which terminate in the *brahmarandra* (cavity of Brahma), which corresponds to the ventricular cavity in the physical body. The ida and pingala nadis also travel upward along the spinal column, but they crisscross each other and the sushumna before terminating in the left and right nostrils, respectively.

The junctions where the ida, pingala, and sushumna nadis

meet along the spinal column are called chakras (wheels). Just as the spokes of a wheel radiate outward from a central hub, so do the other nadis radiate outward from the chakras to other parts of the body. There are seven principal chakras: the *muladhara* chakra at the base of the spine at the level of the pelvic plexus in the physical body, the *svadhishthana* chakra at the level of the hypogastric plexus, the *manipura* chakra at the level of the solar plexus, the *anahata* chakra at the level of the cardiac plexus, the *vishuddha* chakra at the level of the pharangeal plexus, the *ajna* chakra at the level of the nasociliary plexus, and the *sahasrara* chakra at the top of the head. The anterior portion of the sushumna passes through the ajna chakra, and the posterior portion passes behind the skull, the two portions uniting in the brahmarandra.

Yoga anatomy and physiology are clear and accurate to those who systematically study and practice the science of yoga, and they find that it reveals more about the internal functionings of the human body than any modern scientific experiment or explanation. It is true, however, that the ancient descriptions of nadis and chakras bear a remarkable resemblance to modern anatomical descriptions of nerves and plexuses, respectively. Some scientists have tried to establish a correspondence between the two systems, but the assumption behind such an attempt is that the nerves and plexuses belong to the physical body while the nadis and chakras belong to what is known in yoga science as the *sukshma sharira* (subtle body). In other words, they are the subtle counterparts of the nerves and plexuses, respectively. The currents of prana flowing through these nadis are the subtle counterparts of the nerve impulses. The yogis did not dissect the physical body in order to learn about its subtle

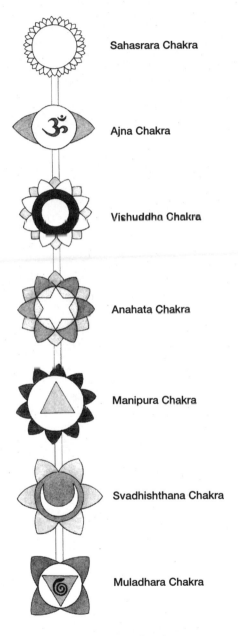

Sahasrara Chakra

Ajna Chakra

Vishuddha Chakra

Anahata Chakra

Manipura Chakra

Svadhishthana Chakra

Muladhara Chakra

The Seven Major Chakras

crosscurrents—dissecting the physical body to look for subtle energies would be futile. They discovered the network of nadis and chakras by mapping the flow of prana through this network, and they developed this mapping ability through introspective experimentation.

The physical body is built around the subtle framework of the nadis and is sustained by the flow of pranic energy through this network. In the average individual, the dynamic and creative aspect of prana is only an infinitesimal fraction of the total energy of prana, the major part of it remaining in a potential, or seed, state. Yoga manuals refer to this latent, stored energy as *kundalini*, which is symbolically represented as a sleeping serpent coiled in the muladhara chakra at the base of the spine. Further, in the average individual, prana flows through ida and pingala, but not through sushumna, this nadi ordinarily being blocked at the base of the spinal column.

The techniques of pranayama are aimed at devitalizing ida and pingala and at the same time opening up sushumna, thus allowing the prana to flow through this middle channel. The yogi then experiences great joy and is freed from the bondage of time, space, and causation. Then, having opened up the sushumna nadi, the yogi rouses the sleeping serpent at the muladhara chakra and guides this tremendous energy upward along sushumna, piercing the six chakras, to the seventh chakra, called the sahasrara, which is represented as a thousand-petaled lotus at the crown of the head. This arousal and ascent of the latent kundalini energy and its merging in the sahasrara is synonymous with the union of *shakti* (cosmic potency) with *shiva* (cosmic consciousness). With this union the yogi achieves liberation from all miseries and bondage. He thus merges his individual soul, *atman,* with the cosmic soul, *Brahman.*

Pranayama is one of the rungs on the ladder of raja yoga. The first four rungs are referred to by some as hatha yoga, or physical yoga, and the last four rungs are known as raja yoga, or the royal path. The first four rungs are *yama* (restraints), *niyama* (observances), *asana* (posture), and *pranayama* (breath control). The four higher rungs are *pratyahara* (sense withdrawal), *dharana* (concentration), *dhyana* (meditation), and *samadhi* (the superconscious state, the ultimate freedom from the cycle of birth and death).

Controlling the breath and calming the nerves is a prerequisite to controlling the mind, and control of the mind is a prerequisite to the ultimate subjugation of the universal energy of prana. To the yogi, body, breath, nerves, mind, prana, and the universe are all part of a continuum, and he does not set up artificial distinctions between them. In Western thinking, however, there has been a much greater tendency for compartmentalization so that, for instance, the sciences of physiology and psychology have maintained their separate identities. Only in recent times have scientists admitted the interrelationship between psyche and soma, and the psychosomatic origins of disease have finally become a valid subject for research and study.

According to yoga and the science of pranayama, disease is a manifestation of an imbalance in the flow of prana. Both body and mind are sustained by prana and thus interact to a greater extent than is normally imagined. For example, scientific experiments have shown that peristalsis (the intestinal churning necessary for digestion) is greatly inhibited by emotions such as anger, fear, and anxiety. Another example of the interrelationship between the body and mind is the influence of emotions on the breath. When we are afraid, breathing becomes shallow and rapid; when depressed, breathing becomes heavy and labored.

Psychologists have shown that there is a correspondence between personality types and breathing patterns. Yoga science also recognizes such a correspondence, but according to yoga, the relationship between the breath and mind is reciprocal. If a certain state of mind results in a certain mode of breathing, then conversely, by consciously adopting that mode of breathing we can evoke the corresponding state of mind. If there is a correspondence between personality type and pattern of breathing, then the yogi states categorically that by changing the pattern of breathing we can transform the personality, for when the mind is disturbed, the breath is disturbed and becomes shallow, rapid, and uneven. By consciously making the breath deep, even, and regular, we will experience a noticeable release of tension and an increased sense of relaxation and tranquility.

Basic Breathing and Cleansing Techniques

Respiration is the most important function of the body. Yet most people are not aware of the simple fact that the breath does not flow equally through the two nostrils. At times one nostril is more active than the other, and at other times it may become less active than the other. This is because on each side of the septum separating the two nostrils, there are structures called turbinates that regulate the pathway of airflow within the inner nose. These turbinates are covered by mucous membrane, which is composed of erectile tissue. The swelling of the turbinates changes the inner configuration of the air pathways and can thus restrict or even block the flow of air. This explains the unequal flow of breath through the nostrils.

One of the aims of yogic breathing techniques is to equalize the airflow in the nostrils. This is a prerequisite for the devitalization of the ida and pingala nadis and the opening up of the blocked sushumna nadi. In a moment, we will consider a breathing technique called *nadi shodhanam,* or purification of the nadis, the practice of which leads to equalization of the breath in the right and left nostrils, and then to the opening of the sushumna nadi. Equalizing the flow of breath calms the mind, and in states of deep meditation this equal flow is evident.

Jala Neti (Water Cleansing)

A preliminary step to equalizing the flow of breath is cleansing the nostrils, and for this yoga manuals describe a technique called *jala neti* (purification with water). Lukewarm water, with a little salt dissolved in it, is poured into one nostril while the head is tilted so as to allow the saline solution to flow out through the other nostril. (A cup can be used to do this, but it is far more convenient to use a pot with a narrow spout.) This lukewarm, saline water not only dissolves and washes away any accumulated mucus and dirt, but it also, by osmosis, draws out excess water from swollen turbinate structures. It also facilitates drainage of the sinuses.

If the water is first poured into the left nostril and flows out through the right, the flow direction is then reversed by pouring the salt water into the right nostril and allowing it to drain through the left. This accomplishes a thorough cleansing of the air passageways. Personal instruction in this technique from a qualified teacher is recommended before attempting it on your own. Daily practice prevents congestion of the sinuses and makes you less susceptible to common colds and other respiratory infections.

Sutra Neti (String Cleansing)

In this exercise a rubber catheter with a cotton string attached is inserted into the nostril and then taken out through the mouth, or string alone may be used if the end has been stiffened with wax. All the implements should be sterilized before they are used and, as has been said before, the demonstration of this technique by a competent teacher is recommended before your first attempt.

This exercise cleanses the nostrils, strengthens the mucous membrane, and benefits the eyes.

Rhythmic Diaphragmatic Breathing

The most important aspect of breath control is diaphragmatic breathing. The average person uses his chest muscles rather than his diaphragm when he breathes, and such breathing is usually shallow, rapid, and irregular. As a consequence, the lower lobes of the lungs, which receive an abundant supply of blood, are not adequately ventilated, so the gas exchange which takes place between the air in the lungs and the blood is inadequate. Respiratory physiologists refer to this as a ventilation-perfusion abnormality. With diaphragmatic breathing, such inequalities between ventilation and perfusion are minimized. There is also evidence to suggest that diaphragmatic breathing is beneficial because it increases the suction pressure created in the thoracic cavity and improves the venous return of blood, thereby reducing the load on the heart and enhancing circulatory function.

Though chest breathing has now become natural and involuntary for most of us, it is really a part of the fight or flight syndrome, aroused when the organism is challenged by some external stress or danger. Because of the reciprocity between the breath and mind, chest breathing, in turn, gives rise to the tension and anxiety associated with the fight or flight syndrome. With chest breathing, the breath is shallow, jerky, and unsteady, resulting in similar unsteadiness of the mind. All techniques aimed at providing relaxation of the body, nerves, and mind will be ineffective unless chest breathing is replaced by deep, even, and steady diaphragmatic breathing.

Although diaphragmatic breathing is simple, easy, and beneficial, the habit of doing it has to be consciously cultivated before it can become automatic. A simple practice to achieve this is to lie on your back on a mat or rug, with one palm placed on the center of the chest and the other on the lower edge of the rib cage where the abdomen begins. As you inhale, the lower edge of the rib cage should expand and the abdomen should rise; as you exhale, the opposite should occur. There should be relatively little movement of the upper chest. By practicing this exercise you will find in due time that diaphragmatic breathing becomes habitual and automatic.

Next you should cultivate the habit of harmonious, rhythmic breathing along with diaphragmatic breathing. Observing the rate of breathing per minute on both inhalation and exhalation is highly therapeutic and is not at all difficult. Breathing between sixteen and twenty breaths per minute is considered average, but when both inhalation and exhalation become slower and smoother, breathing becomes easy.

What is more, modern scientists are aware that during inhalation, plasma from the capillaries oozes into the alveoli (it returns again into the circulation during exhalation), so lengthening the inhalation increases the time available for this transfer to take place. Therefore you should learn to slow down your inhalation first. Rhythmic diaphragmatic breathing also brings more air and oxygen into the air sacs of the lungs and into the bloodstream. It increases the return of venous (oxygen-depleted) blood to the lungs and sends an increased blood supply to the capillaries of the alveoli.

Diaphragmatic breathing can be practiced in a firm standing position, a steady sitting position, or by lying on your back with the hands along the sides of the body, palms upward, and legs slightly apart (this latter position is called *shavasana,* or the corpse posture). Exhalation should be through the nostrils, and there should be no sound in the breath. Having exhaled completely, inhalation begins; minimizing the pause, again breathe through the nostrils, making no sound.

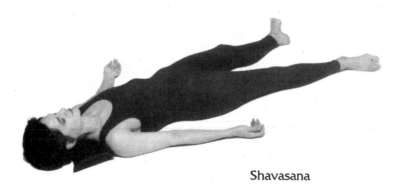

Shavasana

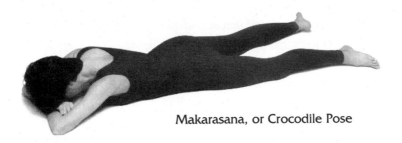

Makarasana, or Crocodile Pose

Makarasana (Crocodile Pose)

If you do not understand or for some reason cannot start practicing diaphragmatic breathing in a sitting position, then start in the crocodile posture. Lie on the stomach, placing the legs a comfortable distance apart and pointing the toes outward. Fold the arms in front of the body, resting the hands on the biceps. Position the arms so that the chest does not touch the floor, and rest the forehead on the arms.

This posture is an excellent teaching device because it allows you to experience how it feels to breathe diaphragmatically, for when you inhale you feel the abdomen pressing against the floor, and when you exhale you feel the abdominal muscles relaxing. So it is easy to note the movement of the diaphragm in this posture.

Sandbag Breathing

This practice will strengthen the abdominal and diaphragmatic muscles. It will also help to regulate the motion of the lungs in cooperation with the movement of the muscles of the diaphragm. Lie on your back in shavasana, seal your lips gently, and relax your body from head to toe. Calm your breath. Now gently place a five-pound sandbag on your abdomen. If you have heart problems, lung problems, or blood pressure abnormalities, place the sandbag on the muscles below the navel, but make sure that no part of the sandbag is supported by the pelvic girdle.

Close your eyes and breathe. Feel how the sandbag rises as you inhale and drops as you exhale. You must make an effort to inhale, but the exhalation should be effortless. After three to five minutes, remove the sandbag and relax on your back for a few more minutes.

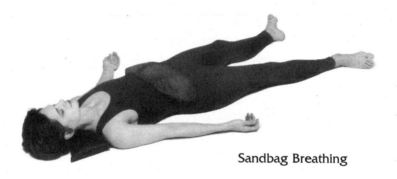

Sandbag Breathing

If you practice regularly, you may want to increase the weight of the sandbag every two weeks. But do this gradually, staying within your comfortable capacity, and do not exceed fifteen pounds.

Diaphragmatic breathing decreases the breath rate considerably. It is the basic exercise that the student practices to accomplish the higher practices and derive benefits from the science of breath.

Breathing air into the deep recesses of the lungs is healthy in all respects. Since the pericardium is attached to the diaphragm, the process of deep breathing causes the diaphragm to descend, stretching the heart downward toward the abdomen. When the lungs are filled with air from the bottom upward, they compress, giving a gentle massage to the heart. As the diaphragm contracts and relaxes, it also massages the heart, liver, and pancreas, and it helps to improve the functions of the spleen, stomach, small intestine, and abdomen as well.

If the practice of rhythmic diaphragmatic breathing is done ten times a day for at least two months, with gradual and equal prolongation of the inhalation and exhalation, the body will experience a sense of deep relaxation and rest—more restful even than the deepest sleep. One will remain free from the stress and strain which is the source of many physical and psychosomatic illnesses. The nerves will be calm, and the voice and face will manifest this serenity. The voice will grow sweeter, and the harsh lines of the face will be replaced by a soft glow.

Nadi Shodhanam (Alternate Nostril Breathing)

Another excellent breathing exercise is called *nadi shodhanam*, which literally means "channel purification."

1. Sit in a calm, quiet, airy place in an easy and steady posture with the head, neck, and trunk erect and in a straight line. The body should be still.

2. Bring the right hand up to the nose; the index and middle fingers should be folded so that the right thumb can be used to close the right nostril and the ring finger used to close the left nostril (Vishnu mudra).

3. With the right nostril closed, exhale completely through the left nostril. The exhalation should be slow, controlled, and free from exertion and jerkiness.

4. At the end of the exhalation, close the left nostril with the ring finger, open the right nostril, and inhale slowly and completely. Inhalation should also be slow, smooth, controlled, and of the same duration as the exhalation.

5. Repeat this cycle of exhalation through the left nostril followed by inhalation through the right nostril two more times.

6. At the end of the third inhalation through the right nostril, exhale completely through the same nostril, still keeping the left nostril closed with the ring finger.

7. At the end of this exhalation close the right nostril and inhale through the left nostril. Repeat this cycle of exhalation through the right nostril followed by inhalation through the left nostril two more times. This completes the exercise.

In summary, the exercise consists of three cycles of exhalation through the left nostril and inhalation through the right nostril, followed by three cycles of exhalation through the right nostril and inhalation through the left nostril.

In the evening, start the exercise with three cycles of exhalation through the right nostril and inhalation through the left nostril, followed by three cycles of exhalation through the left nostril and inhalation through the right nostril. In all phases of this exercise, the exhalation and inhalation should be of equal duration, without a pause between exhalation and inhalation. Breathing should be diaphragmatic and should be slow and controlled, with no sense of exertion. With practice, gradual lengthening of the duration of inhalation and exhalation should be attempted.

There are slight variations on this basic technique in different yoga texts. The student should avoid frequent changes in technique, however, for only with regular practice of the same technique can he reap the full benefits of nadi shodhanam. Further, in some texts retention of the breath between inhalation and exhalation is recommended. This is an advanced form of the exercise and should be attempted only under the guidance of a competent teacher. Otherwise the student may harm himself irreparably. Under proper guidance retention may be practiced, the period of retention being gradually increased so long as it does not in any way affect the rhythm, evenness, and equality of inhalation and exhalation. The recommended ratio between the durations of inhalation, retention, and exhalation is 1:4:2. After mastering the retention of breath after inhalation, the student attempts retention after exhalation, again by gradually increasing the length of time the breath is held.

Pranayama is a highly developed and complex science, and the advanced techniques require expert guidance. They should not be attempted purely on the basis of instructions found in books. Unless one has the prerequisites for such advanced techniques, more harm than good will result, for the aspirant will have awakened the energies of prana to a degree that is beyond his capacity to contain and control.

The basic form of nadi shodhanam without retention, described above, and a few other types of pranayama may be practiced safely, based on the instructions given here. But to repeat: retention of breath does require the sanction and guidance of a teacher well-versed in pranayama.

Kapalabhati Pranayama (Shining Face Breathing)

Kapalabhati literally means "the pranayama that makes the forehead and entire face lustrous." It helps clean the sinuses and all other respiratory passages, and it stimulates the

abdominal muscles and digestive organs. A sense of exhila-
ration is experienced with this practice.

This exercise consists of a vigorous and forceful expulsion
of breath, using the diaphragm and abdominal muscles, followed by a relaxation of the abdominal muscles, resulting in
a slow, passive inhalation. This cycle of an active and vigorous exhalation followed by a passive inhalation is repeated
several times in quick succession. In the beginning you can
attempt between seven and twenty-one cycles, depending on
your capacity.

Bhastrika Pranayama (Bellows Breathing)

The word *bhastrika* means "bellows." In this pranayama
the abdominal muscles work like bellows. The beneficial effects of this exercise are similar to those of kapalabhati.

In this exercise, the diaphragm and abdominal muscles
are employed as in kapalabhati, but here both inhalation
and exhalation are vigorous and forceful. Between seven
and twenty-one cycles may be attempted, according to your
capacity, and the cycles should follow each other in quick
succession.

Ujjayi Pranayama (Victorious Breathing)

The word *ujjayi* may be interpreted as "control or victory
arising from a process of expansion." This pranayama en-
hances the ventilation of the lungs, removes phlegm, calms
the nerves, and fills the whole body with vitality.

Inhalation and exhalation during ujjayi are slow and deep,
and they take place with partial closure of the glottis. This
produces a sound like sobbing, but it is even and continuous. During inhalation, the incoming air is felt on the roof
of the palate and is accompanied by the sibilant sound *sa*.
During exhalation, the outgoing air is felt on the roof of the

palate and is accompanied by the aspirate sound *ha*. During inhalation, the abdominal muscles are kept slightly contracted, and during exhalation, abdominal pressure is exerted until the breath is completely expelled.

Bhramari Pranayama (Bee Breathing)

A *bhramari* is a large bee. The sound of the buzzing of a bee is made during exhalation in this exercise. Inhale completely through both nostrils. Exhaling as in ujjayi, produce the humming sound of a bee. Repeat for two to three minutes. Bhramari soothes the nerves and calms the mind.

Sitali Pranayama (Hissing Breath I)

Sitali and *sitkari* both are exercises for cooling and soothing the body. Curl the tongue lengthwise until it resembles a tube (those who cannot do this should practice sitkari instead). Let the tip of the tongue protrude outside the lips. Inhaling, make a hissing sound with the breath. Exhale completely through both nostrils. Repeat three times.

Sitkari Pranayama (Hissing Breath II)

Roll the tongue back as far as possible toward the soft palate. Let the lips part, and clench the teeth. Inhaling through the teeth, make a hissing sound with the breath. Exhale completely through both nostrils. Repeat three times.

The following exercises *(surya bhedana, murccha, and plavini)* are described here to illustrate important yogic breathing techniques. These three, however, should only be practiced under the guidance of a qualified teacher. An experienced teacher can show the student how to avoid damaging the heart and lungs during the procedure.

Surya Bhedana Pranayama

In this exercise, the breath is inhaled through the right nostril, retained, and then exhaled through the left nostril.

Murccha Pranayama

Inhale completely through both nostrils. Apply the chin lock, and then slowly and gently exhale.

Plavini Pranayama

Plavini is one of the most advanced pranayama exercises. In this practice, the stomach is first filled completely with air. Then, while the air remains in the stomach, the lungs are filled completely. The breath is retained, and then finally exhaled. This method of inhalation, retention, and exhalation is repeated the desired number of times, and when the exercise is finished, the air is regurgitated through the mouth.

There are a few, more rare, advanced pranayama exercises which are meant exclusively for adept yogis. Such exercises are traditionally imparted to advanced students by their preceptors.

Patanjali, the codifier of the *Yoga Sutra,* while explaining various ways of bringing the mind under control, also includes the method of pranayama. The whole secret of the science of breath lies in the interpretation of sutra 1.34. Here Patanjali uses different words for inhalation, exhalation, and retention. According to him, having control over the pause in the breath is called pranayama. This means that to control, eliminate, and expand the pause is pranayama. In Sanskrit the pause is called *kumbhaka.* Hence, sutra 1.34 is an aphorism, a brief note which the competent teacher can explain to his students. Actually, *pranayama* in practice means "pause," though various authors have tried to explain it in other ways. All the breathing exercises are meant to control, eliminate, and expand that pause.

Hatha yoga manuals mention eight varieties of kumb-haka. It is a practical subject, and competent yogis alone know the secrets of the nature of the pause. The kumbhakas should be practiced carefully under a competent guide, never by reading manuals alone. Nor should they be practiced without applying the *bandhas* (locks).

Bandhas and Their Application

All aspirants are strictly advised not to practice the exercises of kumbhaka (retention of breath) without applying the bandhas. Bandhas are locks, and there are three of them: *jalandhara* bandha (the chin lock), *uddiyana* bandha (the abdominal lock), and *mula* bandha (the anal lock).

Jalandhara Bandha (Chin Lock)

The internal and external carotid arteries, which bring the blood supply to the brain, lie on both sides of the neck. When pressure is applied to these arteries through the chin lock, the nerve impulses traveling to the brain attenuate body consciousness and bring about a trancelike condition. This stimulation also slows down the heart, and the *vijnani nadi*, which can be translated as "channel of consciousness," can thus be brought under conscious control. It is said in the *Shiva Samhita* that by putting pressure on the carotid sinus nerves, a blissful state of mind is experienced. In other words, when the chin lock is practiced, both in exhalation and inhalation, control of the vijnani nadi becomes easy. But it takes a long time—sometimes years—for the yogi to gain mastery of the jalandhara bandha.

When the chin lock is not applied after the retention of the breath, the air wants to rush out after deep inhalation, even if the glottis is kept closed. So it rushes through the auditory

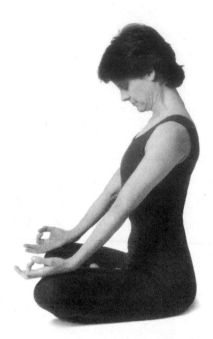

Jalandhara Bandha

tubes and disturbs the inner ear, causing various disorders. Therefore jalandhara bandha is applied to prevent such disorders. The glottis is first closed; then, by proper application of the chin lock, practicing khumbhaka becomes easy.

A few doctors in India put pressure on the carotid arteries and thus give yogic anesthesia to the patient. They even perform minor surgery with this "anesthetic." The same principle has been adopted by martial art experts, especially in the school of kung fu. Children often experience that pleasant feeling of "passing out" when they unconsciously learn to put pressure on the carotid artery. Through jalandhara bandha, yogis bring about conscious control of this phenomenon and thus attain a state of joy before meditating.

Uddiyana Bandha (Abdominal Lift)

Uddiyana is an exercise which involves the diaphragm, ribs, and abdominal muscles, and it can be practiced either standing or sitting in one of the meditative postures. In the standing position, place the feet approximately two feet apart. Keep the spine straight, bend the knees slightly, and lean forward from the waist far enough to place the palms of the hands just above the knees. Exhale completely, and place the chin on the hollow of the throat. Without inhaling, suck the abdominal muscles in and up, pulling the navel toward the spine. This motion pulls the diaphragm up and creates a cavity on the front side of the abdomen under the rib cage. The back will curve slightly. This position is held for as long as it remains comfortable. Then slowly inhale and relax.

Never force the abdominal muscles outward; use force only in pulling the muscles in and upward. Do not practice this exercise if there is any problem with high blood pressure, hiatal hernia, ulcers, or heart disorders. Women should not practice it during menstruation or pregnancy. Uddiyana is one of the finest exercises for the abdominal organs.

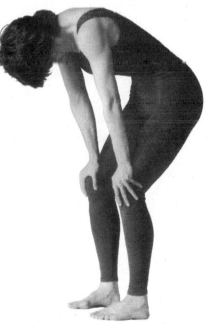

Uddiyana Bandha

Mula Bandha (Anal Lock)

Mula bandha (the anal lock) is an exercise in which the sphincter muscles are contracted. Both the external and the internal sphincter muscles are contracted and then held. This bandha is used during pranayama and meditation.

Mudras

Mudra means "seal." There are a number of mudras mentioned in the yoga texts including *maha* mudra, *khecari* mudra, *ashvini* mudra, *yoga* mudra, *vajroli* mudra, *jnana* mudra, *Vishnu* mudra, and others.

One mudra used during meditation is jnana mudra (the finger lock). Once the student has arranged his feet and legs and has placed his body in a comfortable sitting posture, it is important that the arms, hands, and fingers be arranged accordingly so that they do not become a source of distraction. Jnana mudra is then applied. Although there are various ways of placing the fingers, the simplest is to place the thumb and the forefinger

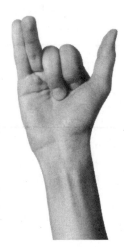

Vishnu Mudra

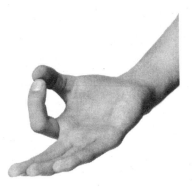

Jnana Mudra

together and rest the hands, palms downward, on the knees. Vishnu mudra, which is used during pranayama exercises, is described in the nadi shodhanam section.

The Importance of Breath Awareness in Meditation

Breath awareness is an essential part of meditation. Authentic schools of meditation teach breath awareness before leading a student toward advanced techniques of meditation, but some of the modern schools have failed to grasp its significance. This is why their teachers are unable to lead their students to deeper states of meditation.

The mind is in the habit of identifying itself with the objects of the world, and it does not become aware of internal states as long as it remains in this dissipated condition. With systematic discipline, however, the mind starts traveling inward toward the more subtle levels of consciousness, and when one attains a state of perfect stillness and tranquility, that which is beyond the mind reveals itself.

In learning to meditate, tranquility of mind is an important factor, but even more important is breath awareness. The primary step is to find a steady, comfortable, and easy posture. The second step is to develop calm, serene, and even breathing. The third is to calm and steady the mind, which is the only means for experiencing the deeper levels of being. The fourth step is to gain control of the conscious mind, for this control can make one dynamic and creative. In the fifth step, the involuntary system as well as a vast part of the unconscious mind, including the memory, are brought under conscious control, and in the sixth step, the mind becomes aware that it is conditioned by time, space, and causation. Through meditation, the mind can be trained to remain aware of the present moment, the door to eternity. In the seventh step, constant awareness is developed through the regular practice of meditation, and the highest state of *turiya* is attained. This state is full of bliss, peace, happiness, and wisdom.

After serious observation and analysis of its functionings, yogis have found that the mind forms the habit of being conditioned, either by remembering past experiences or by imagining the future. There is no technique which helps it to become aware of the present except that of meditation and contemplation. But meditation is not a method of allowing the mind to roam aimlessly. It is a conscious effort of coordinating the body, the breath, and the mind. In the monastic tradition, teachers do not teach the advanced techniques of meditation unless they see the signs and symptoms of stillness of the body and serenity of the breath developing in the student.

When a student learns to still his body, he becomes aware of many tremors, twitchings, and movements that he was not conscious of before. Since childhood he has learned to move, but no one has taught him how to be still, and sitting still is very important, for the less movement there is in the body, the steadier the mind will be. All of the tremors of the body are caused by an undisciplined and untrained mind. When a student examines his behavior, he finds that not a single act or gesture is independent. The mind moves first, and then the body moves—and the more the body moves, the more the mind dissipates. When the student has learned to be still, however, and begins practicing the techniques of breath awareness and meditation, he discovers that he can have conscious control over his body, breath, and mind.

So the first thing one must learn is to sit still. The right posture is one that makes one steady and comfortable, and it is one in which all or most of the body parts are free from the pressure of other body parts.

Sukhasana (Easy Pose)

Sitting with the head, neck, and trunk straight, place the left foot beneath the right knee and the right foot beneath the left knee. Each knee rests on the opposite foot. Place the hands on the corresponding knees and apply the finger lock. This is a posture for beginners.

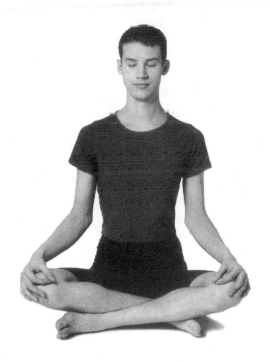

Sukhasana, or Easy Pose

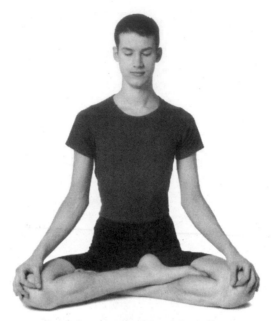

Svastikasana, or Auspicious Pose

Svastikasana (Auspicious Pose)

In ancient times, the svastika was a symbol of divine blessings. In this posture, the heels and ankle bones are not aligned. Bend the left leg at the knee and place the sole of the left foot against the right thigh. Place the right foot on top of the left calf, and put the outer edge of the foot and the toes between the thigh and calf muscles. The big toe should be visible. Pull the toes of the left foot between the right thigh and calf so that the big toe is visible. Place the hands on the corresponding knees, joining the fingers in the finger lock.

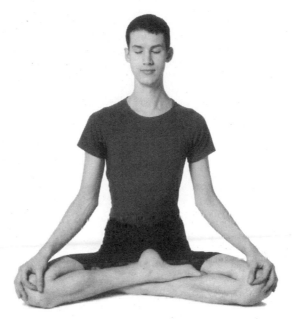

Siddhasana, or Accomplished Pose

Siddhasana (Accomplished Pose)

A favorite of yogis, siddhasana is called the accomplished posture, or the posture of adepts. In it advanced yogis meditate for hours and hours at a time or practice advanced pranayama techniques. Place the left heel at the perineum and the right heel at the pubic bone above the organ of generation. Arrange the feet and legs so that the ankles are in one line or touch one another. Place the toes of the right foot between the left thigh and calf so that only the big toe is visible. Pull the toes of the left foot up between the right thigh and calf so the big toe is visible. This is the finest of all postures, but it could be uncomfortable for those who are not advanced.

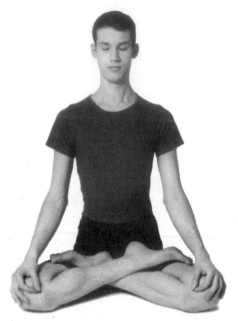

Padmasana, or Lotus Pose

Padmasana (Lotus Pose)

Padma means "lotus." It is a symbol of yoga because just as the lotus grows in the water but keeps its petals untouched by the water, so does the yogi live in the world and yet remain above. Immense benefits are derived from this posture. To do it you should take your place firmly on a cushion (or a fourfolded blanket or a pillow). Bend the left leg at the knee joint; turn up the sole and place the foot firmly at the right groin. Similarly, fold the right leg, turning up the sole and placing it firmly at the left groin. Both heels should press firmly against the abdominal wall. Place the hands on the corresponding knees and assume jnana mudra (the finger lock). Applying bandhas or locks in this posture is complicated, and without expert guidance they should not be applied. Applying bandhas in padmasana for a long time definitely disturbs the intestinal movement and creates gastric problems. As an exercise, however, it is one of the finest for the abdominal muscles.

Maitri Asana (Friendship Pose)

For a modern man it is sometimes more convenient to sit on a straight-backed wooden chair, keeping the head, neck, and trunk straight and placing the hands on the knees. The legs should not be crossed but firmly placed on the ground. Buddhist scriptures describe this posture.

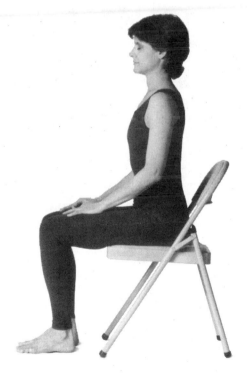

Maitri Asana, or Friendship Pose

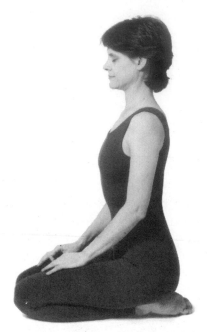

Vajrasana, or Kneeling Pose

Vajrasana (Kneeling Pose)

Sit in a kneeling position with the head, neck, and trunk straight. Rest the hands, palms downward, above the knees. This posture is mostly practiced in non-yogic traditions such as Zen and the Islamic tradition. It can also be used for meditation, but if it is continued for a long time, it can sometimes cause pulled muscles by overstretching the ligaments of the foot.

Having attained a comfortable, stable, and easy posture, the student will then be able to become aware of his breath. Breath awareness is a reliable guide for experiencing the higher level of consciousness and for making the mind one-pointed. It prepares the meditator for applying sushumna.

Although the word *sushumna* cannot be translated into English, according to me, it means the state of mind that is undisturbed and joyous, and which occurs when the breath starts flowing freely and smoothly through both nostrils. Such a mental condition is necessary in order for the mind to travel into deeper levels of consciousness, for if the mind is not brought to a state of joy, it cannot remain steady, and an unsteady mind is not at all fit for meditation. Another school of yoga, which teaches the awakening of kundalini, says that without awakening sushumna, deep meditation and the awakening of kundalini are impossible. There are only three techniques for applying sushumna: concentrating on the bridge between the two nostrils; doing pranayama breathing exercises while applying jalandhara bandha; and meditating on the chakra system.

The process of awakening sushumna is possible only when a student starts enjoying being still. When he sits in a calm, quiet place in a comfortable, steady posture, and when body tremors are not a source of disturbance, he can start meditating on the flow of breath. The moment he does, he becomes aware of four irregularities in the breath: shallowness, jerks, noise, and that which disturbs him the most, the pause between inhalation and exhalation.

Much has been spoken about this pause in the scriptures, but practice makes one increasingly aware of its importance. When a student starts meditating on the flow of breath the pause distracts his mind. Some of the scriptures say that the pause can be expanded; some say it can be omitted. In the beginning, however, one has to go through the exercises of pranayama and later the exercises of breath retention under the guidance of a competent teacher. Those who do not want to do pranayama exercises can still do meditation, but without breath awareness a deep state of meditation is impossible.

In breath awareness, the duration of inhalation and exhalation is carefully judged mentally, and the mind closely and intimately follows the movement of the breath. Here lies the difference between breathing exercises and breath awareness. In breathing exercises, one is taught to keep a count of the amount of air inhaled and exhaled, but in breath awareness it is done mentally only. No fingers are used to close the nostrils. Through breath awareness, the power of attention is strengthened, and attention is the very key to meditation. In breath awareness, there is no external distraction, and attention is not dissipated. We are not discussing breathing exercises here—breath awareness is an advanced technique; it truly comes after one has practiced the various exercises of breathing described earlier. Breath awareness is vital for a student who wants to learn the higher techniques of meditation.

The breath is a bridge between body and mind. Advanced yogis observe that the breath is like a thermometer which registers the conditions of the mind and the influence of the external environment on the body. Those who have studied their breath behavior also know their mental and physical behavior. Their lives are guided by their control of *svaras* (life ripples).

The behavior of the breath can also warn of illness. For example, when the body suffers from fever, the nostrils start behaving in an unusual way. One of them, for instance, may either start flowing excessively or become blocked for an extended period. In such a condition, the respiratory system does not function normally; the lungs, heart, and related systems are disturbed, and the mind loses its equilibrium. Advanced yogis use their breath behavior to watch the capacity of their mind and body, and they control the behavior of their breath by various exercises.

The breath and the mind are interdependent. If one retains the breath, his mind starts becoming one-pointed; if the breath is irregular and jerky, the mind is dissipated. After attaining a steady posture, meditation on the breath, or breath awareness, is natural.

Breath awareness strengthens the mind and makes it easier for it to become inward. When the mind starts following the flow of the breath, one becomes aware of the reality that all the creatures of the world are breathing the same breath. There is a direct communication between the student and that center of the cosmos which supplies breath to all living creatures. This is a living philosophy. As long as the center, or living unit in human life, receives prana (vital force) through the breath, the body/mind relationship is sustained. When this communication is disrupted, the conscious mind fails and the body is separated from the inner unit of life. This separation is called death.

Various schools recommend different objects for making the mind one-pointed. These are both concrete and abstract; for example, they can be sound syllables, mantras, or images, but none of these objects is helpful in the long run without breath awareness. It is advisable for beginners to develop the habit of breath awareness and not to worry about any other kind of object for the mind to rest upon, for breath awareness is a most natural and essential step for attaining the higher state of meditation.

Meditation is the sustained state of one-pointedness of mind. In deep meditation, the one-pointed mind is able to pierce through the layers of the conscious and unconscious minds to the superconscious state. This breakthrough is called samadhi. On achieving it, one is freed from all bondage and transcends the limitations of time, space, and causation. The microcosm expands to become the macrocosm, just as a drop of water merges with the ocean and becomes the ocean. The individual atman is united with, and achieves total identity with, the cosmic Brahman. Such a one has found the kingdom of God within himself and has won the ultimate freedom—freedom from the endless chain of birth and death. The evolution of man to God is now complete.

RECOMMENDATIONS FOR FURTHER STUDY

The following will be especially helpful in advancing your understanding and practice of yoga and meditation:

Diet and Nutrition . . . . Rudolph M. Ballentine, M.D.

Meditation and Its Practice . . . . Swami Rama

Path of Fire and Light, Volume I . . . . . . Swami Rama

The Royal Path: Practical Lessons on Yoga
(formerly *Lectures on Yoga*) . . . . Swami Rama

Superconscious Meditation . . Usharbudh Arya, D. Litt.

Yoga and Psychotherapy . . . . . . Swami Rama, Rudolph
 Ballentine, M.D., and Swami Ajaya, Ph.D.

Yoga: Mastering the Basics . . . . . Sandra Anderson and
 Rolf Sovik, Psy.D.

You may also find several relaxation and meditation tapes to be useful, including:

Guided Meditation for Beginners

A Guide to Intermediate Meditation

First Step Toward Advanced Meditation

Learn to Meditate

31 and 61 Points

These and other books and tapes on meditation are available from the Himalayan Institute Press. For a catalog or further information, call 800-822-4547 or 717-253-5551, e-mail: hibooks@himalayaninstitute.org, or fax: 717-251-7812.

INDEX

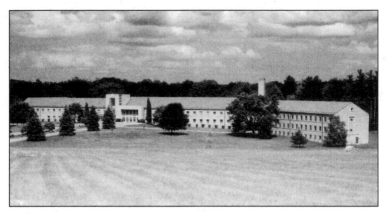

The main building of the Institute headquarters, near Honesdale, Pennsylvania.

THE HIMALAYAN INSTITUTE

Founded in 1971 by Swami Rama, the Himalayan Institute has been dedicated to helping people grow physically, mentally, and spiritually by combining the best knowledge of both the East and the West.

Our international headquarters is located on a beautiful 400-acre campus in the rolling hills of the Pocono Mountains of northeastern Pennsylvania. The atmosphere here is one to foster growth, increased inner awareness, and calm. Our grounds provide a wonderfully peaceful and healthy setting for our seminars and extended programs. Students from around the world join us here to attend programs in such diverse areas as hatha yoga, meditation, stress reduction, Ayurveda, nutrition, Eastern philosophy, psychology, and other subjects. Whether the programs are for weekend meditation retreats, week-long seminars on spirituality, months-long residential programs, or holistic health services, the attempt here is to provide an environment of gentle inner progress. We invite you to join with us in the ongoing process of personal growth and development.

The Institute is a nonprofit organization. Your membership in the Institute helps to support its programs. Please call or write for information on becoming a member.

Institute Programs, Services, and Facilities

Institute programs share an emphasis on conscious holistic living and personal self-development, including:

- Special weekend or extended seminars to teach skills and techniques for increasing your ability to be healthy and enjoy life
- Meditation retreats and advanced meditation and philosophical instruction
- Vegetarian cooking and nutritional training
- Hatha yoga workshops
- Hatha yoga teacher training
- Residential programs for self-development
- Holistic health services and Ayurvedic Rejuvenation Programs through the Institute's Center for Health and Healing.

A *Quarterly Guide to Programs and Other Offerings* is free within the USA. To request a copy, or for further information, call 800-822-4547 or 570-253-5551, fax 570-253-9078, email bqinfo@himalayaninstitute.org, write the Himalayan Institute, RR 1 Box 1127, Honesdale, PA 18431-9706 USA or visit our website at www.himalayaninstitute.org.

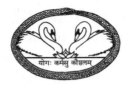

THE HIMALAYAN INSTITUTE PRESS

The Himalayan Institute Press has long been regarded as "The Resource for Holistic Living." We publish dozens of titles, as well as audio and video tapes, that offer practical methods for living harmoniously and achieving inner balance. Our approach addresses the whole person—body, mind, and spirit—integrating the latest scientific knowledge with ancient healing and self-development techniques.

As such, we offer a wide array of titles on physical and psychological health and well-being, spiritual growth through meditation and other yogic practices, as well as translations of yogic scriptures.

Our yoga accessories include the Japa Kit for meditation practice, the Neti™ Pot, the ideal tool for sinus and allergy sufferers, and The Breath Pillow,™ a unique tool for learning health-supportive diaphragmatic breathing.

Subscriptions are available to a bimonthly magazine, *Yoga International*, which offers thought-provoking articles on all aspects of meditation and yoga, including yoga's sister science, Ayurveda.

For a free catalog call 800-822-4547 or 570-253-5551, email hibooks@himalayaninstitute.org, fax 570-253-6360, write the Himalayan Institute Press, RR 1 Box 1129, Honesdale, PA 18431-9709 USA or visit our website at www.himalayaninstitute.org.

ABOUT SWAMI RAMA

Born in 1925 in northern India, Swami Rama was raised from early childhood by a great Bengali yogi and saint who lived in the foothills of the Himalayas. In his youth he practiced the various disciplines of yoga science and philosophy in the traditional monasteries of the Himalayas and studied with many spiritual adepts, including Mahatma Gandhi, Sri Aurobindo, and Rabindranath Tagore. He also traveled to Tibet to study with his grandmaster.

He received his higher education at Prayaga, Varanasi, and Oxford University, England. At the age of twenty-four he became Shankaracharya of Karvirpitham in South India, the highest spiritual position in India. During this term he had a tremendous impact on the spiritual customs of that time: he dispensed with useless formalities and rituals, made it possible for all segments of society to worship in the temples, and encouraged the instruction of women in meditation. He renounced the dignity and prestige of this high office in 1952 to return to the Himalayas to intensify his yogic practices.

After completing an intense meditative practice in the cave monasteries, he emerged with the determination to serve humanity, particularly to bring the teachings of the East to the West. With the encouragement of his master, Swami Rama began his task by studying Western philosophy and psychology. He worked as a medical consultant in London and assisted in parapsychological research in Moscow. He then returned to India, where he established an ashram in Rishikesh. He completed his degree in homeopathy at the medical college in Darbhanga in 1960. He came to the United States in 1969, bringing his knowledge and wisdom to the West. His teachings combine Eastern spirituality with modern Western therapies.

Swami Rama came to America upon the invitation of Dr. Elmer Green of the Menninger Foundation of Topeka, Kansas, as a consultant in a research project investigating the voluntary control of involuntary states. He participated in experiments that helped to revolutionize scientific thinking about the relationship between body and mind, amazing scientists by his demonstrating, under laboratory conditions, precise conscious control of autonomic physical responses and mental functioning, feats previously thought to be impossible.

Swami Rama founded the Himalayan International Institute of Yoga Science and Philosophy, the Himalayan Institute Hospital Trust in India, and many centers throughout the world. He is the author of numerous books on health, meditation, and the yogic scriptures. Swami Rama left his body in November 1996.

ABOUT RUDOLPH BALLENTINE, M.D.

Rudolph Ballentine, M.D., is a respected leader in the field of alternative and complementary medicine. A graduate of Duke University Medical School, he was appointed to the faculty of the department of psychiatry at Louisiana State University School of Medicine. He was a post graduate fellow in Ayurvedic medicine in India, and has also studied homeopathy in India and psychology in the U.S. and France.

Dr. Ballentine directed the Himalayan Institute's Combined Therapy Department for more than fifteen years under the guidance of the founder of the Institute, Sri Swami Rama. He is the co-author of *Yoga and Psychotherapy* and has written and edited a number of related works, such as *The Theory and Practice of Meditation* and *Joints and Glands Exercises*. Dr. Ballentine is the author of *Radical Healing, Transition to Vegetarianism*, and *Diet and Nutrition: A Holistic Approach*, which has sold over 100,000 copies. He is currently the director of the Center for Holistic Medicine in New York City.

ABOUT ALAN HYMES, M.D.

Alan Hymes, M.D., is a cardiovascular and thoracic sur-
geon. A pioneer in the field of breath research, he has
studied the interrelationship between breathing patterns and
cardiovascular disease.